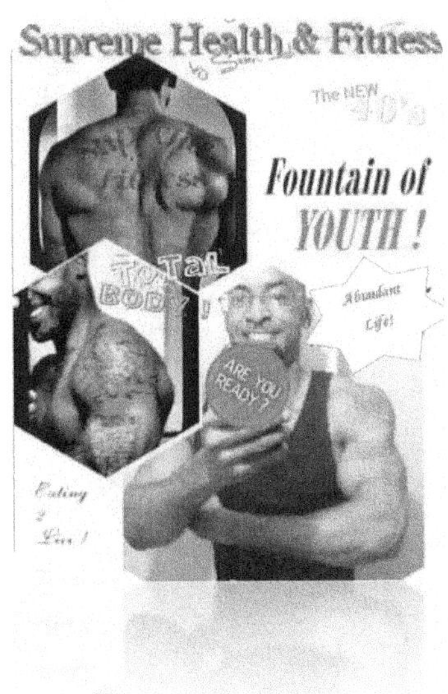

I0789805

Handbook To Supreme Health & Fitness!

*At-Home Guide to Successfully Build Your God-Body!

Supreme Health
Staff & Scientist:

Kareem Tyree
Khalil Malik

Gabriella Monique
Sean Ali

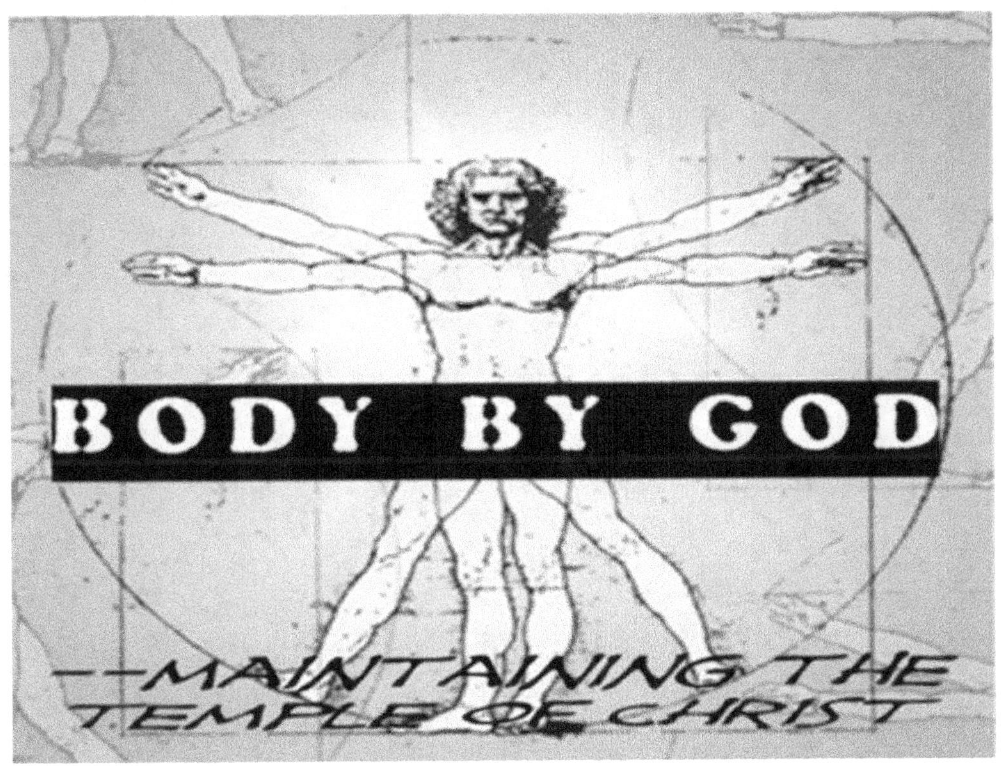
BODY BY GOD
—MAINTAINING THE TEMPLE OF CHRIST

Supreme Health & Fitness by Sean Ali!

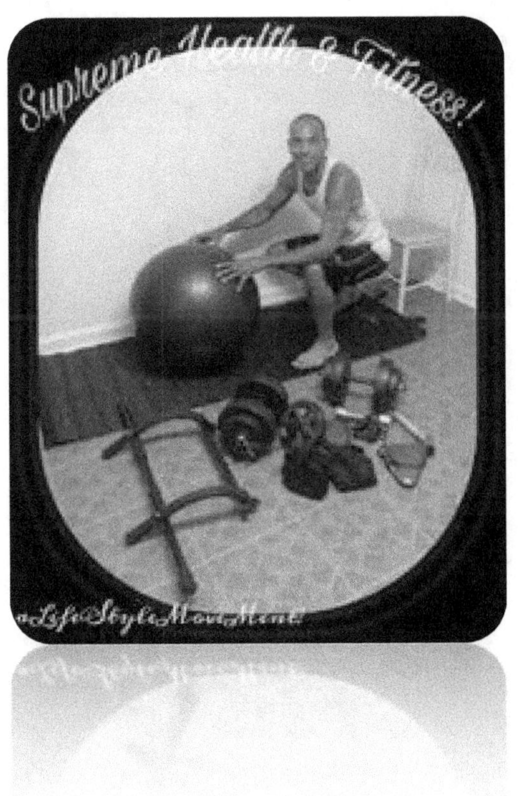

Achieving and Maintaining Supreme Health by Increasing the level of and Knowledge Science of Life!

Supreme Health & Fitness!

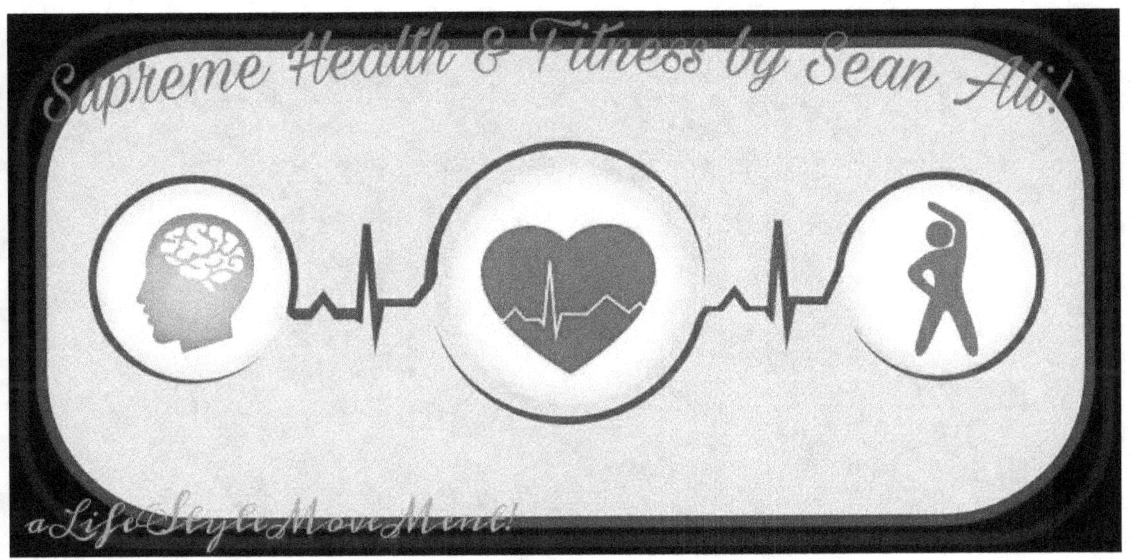

Table of Contents

*****

TAKE CARE OF YOUR BODY. IT'S THE ONLY PLACE YOU HAVE TO LIVE IN.

Introduction

Peace and Blessings of LIFE!

This HandBook represents Volume 4 of the Abundant Life Series, wherein we Strive to Create the God-Body that will Successfully carry us INTO the Enjoyment of Abundant LIFE!

I begin this book with the 2 simple questions:

- *Do YOU want to Improve the Quality of YOUR Life?*
- *Do YOU want to Experience and Enjoy Abundant Life?*

***** THEN THIS BOOK IS FOR YOU!!! *****

In this small HandBook we focus on 2 particular areas of Supreme Health – Flexibility and Muscular Development ... Both of which can very easily be performed At-Home or anywhere that You happen to be.

The more Flexible you are the better Range-of-Motion you can achieve, your Balance is improved and more stable, you experience Less Muscle Tension and Crams.

The Main Benefit of Flexibility is Your Increase in Power and the Ability to Heal, Recover and Maintain Your God-Body!

Practice Creates Perfection ... in the is HandBook are Activities that help Us Practice Abundant Life ... Therefore, You Grow INTO Perfection of Abundant Life ... Leading to the Enjoyment of Abundant LIFE!!!

Life is Energy and we are Energy-based Life forms. The lack-of Energy is the state of being that we call DEATH!

The Science of Flexibility is HOW we keep the Awesome Body limber and the Muscle and Tissue fabric easily conditioned and ready to Receive and Utilize the Life Energy. Dis-eases, Pain, Sicknesses, and Death are all by-products of lack-of Life Energy and/or the in-ability of it to continue to Flow Through US!

Both Flexibility and Exercise are can both be applied MENTALLY as well as Physically!

As we perform these Activities with our Bodies, I have introduced Mental Activities to coincide with the physical motion ... So as You are Building Your God-Body, Your simultaneously Creating the Mental abilities and environment necessary to Achieve Abundant Life!

Abundant Life first Begins as a Mental Process ... an Idea that we can Envision OurSelves 100, 200, 500 years from now ... still Very Healthy, Vibrant and full of Youthful Exuberance!!!!!!

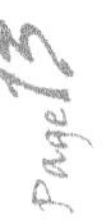

One of the main purposes of exercise is to Improve and Maintain our Awesome Gift from the Creator – God-Body, so that it can Successfully carry us into the Enjoyment of Abundant LIFE.

The main way exercise accomplishes this is by creating the right amount of Pressure, Force and Stress (the Good kind) on the body so that it will increase Oxygen (Breath of LIFE) intake.

The 2nd is by keeping the God-Body In-Shape and Toned.!

Exercise is not meant to have us develop excessive and abnormally huge muscles. Being over-weight or obese have the SAME health Problems. The only difference is the Obesity is from Fat alone and Over-Weight is from Muscles or Fat. Both are equally Dangerous and neither offers a long or enjoyable Lifestyle or LIFE-Span.

In this HandBook we focus on the exercises that help Strengthen your God-Body, with particular emphasis on everyday movements and Muscle Systems. They are designed to show you just How EASY it is to Build and Maintain Your Own Supreme Health .... In the COMFORT and SAFETY of Your Own Home!!!!

When we exercise it's like renewing or winding-up our Energy and even though we can be exhausted at the end, we gain significantly more Energy than we use.

Our ability to Heal ourselves, our Immune System and even Digestion (as well as almost all of our Organs and Systems) Benefit from daily Exercise.

Just imagine that as little as 30 minutes a day of exercise or other physical activities can be the Preventive measure we need to ensure that we never get sick.

Within these 30 minutes we can use or burn any negative elements that may be inside of Self and be potential harmful.

Within this 30 minutes is the catalyst between Youthful Exuberance and Old Age!

30 minutes is the MINIMUM amount of daily exercise recommended to maintain a state of Health. NOW Increase this 30 minutes to 60 MINUTES!

That's DOUBLED the benefits and a significant Increase in Life Energy and the ability to Successfully Enjoy Abundant Life!

Abundant Life is a GIFT from the Creator!

We are Created In the Image and Likeness of The CREATOR. When YOU look at YOURSELF = YOU SEE GOD!

When YOU Look at YOUR Body = YOU SEE A GOD-BODY!

Open this Handbook and let's Create the God-Body that will Successfully carry You INTO the Enjoyment of Abundant Life!!

Peace!

Sean Ali

OR DO YOU NOT KNOW THAT **YOUR BODY IS A TEMPLE** OF THE HOLY SPIRIT WITHIN YOU, WHOM YOU HAVE FROM GOD? YOU ARE NOT YOUR OWN, FOR YOU WERE BOUGHT WITH A PRICE. SO GLORIFY GOD IN YOUR BODY.

1 CORINTHIANS 6:19-20

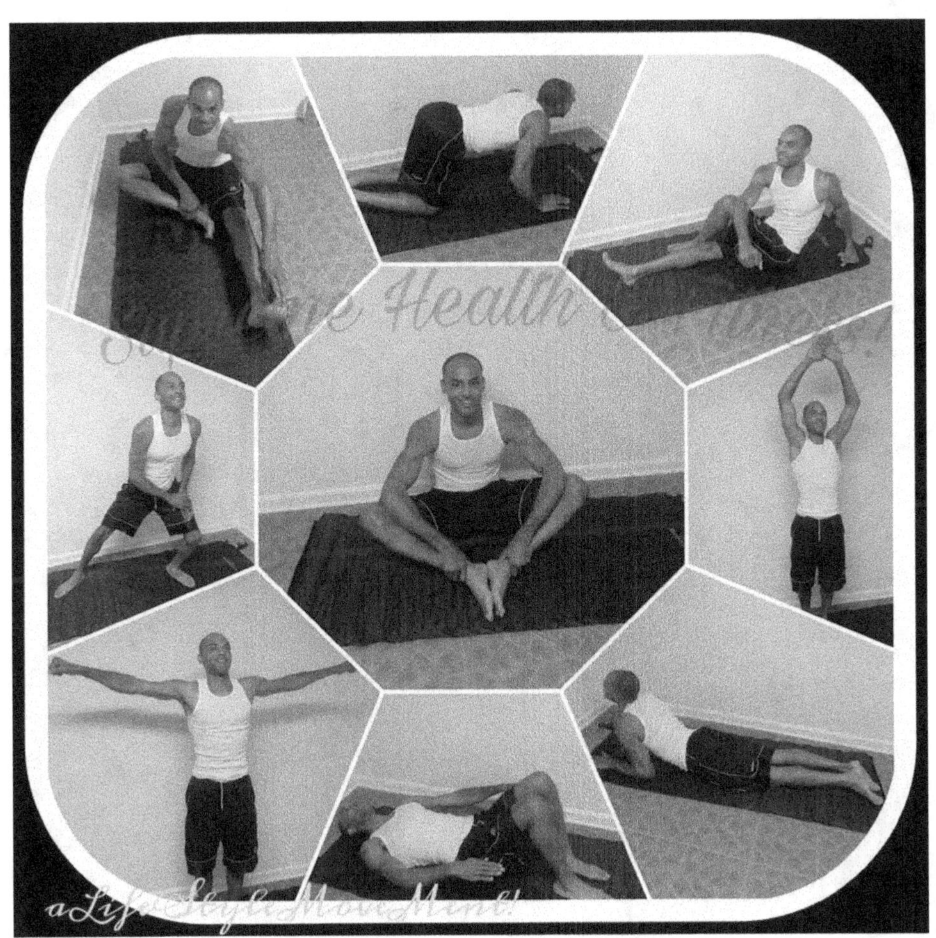

Creating Your Flexibility

*****

What Determines Flexibility?

Flexibility is the ability of a Joint and its surrounding Muscle to move through their full **range of motion**. Flexibility significantly Improves our ability to Move and perpetually sustain our Motion. We are born with Incredible Flexibility and it is only through lack-of use as we age that we lose our Vital Flexibility.

■ **Flexibility** is an important part of physical fitness, but it is often overlooked during workouts.

■ **Flexibility** is achieved by **Stretching**. Stress causes muscles to contract and tighten. Stretching helps muscles relax, relieving pain from muscular stress.

■ There are two recommended kinds of stretching: **Static** and **Dynamic**.

Physiology of Stretching

Areas within your **Muscles** and **Tendons** protect them from **over-stretching** or **tearing** during a quick stretch by creating a stretch reflex. For example, someone tapping your leg just below the kneecap quickly stretches the quadriceps muscle. This makes your thigh contract and kick out your lower leg. **The Quicker the Stretch, the Stronger the Reflex.**

The **protective action** of Tendons causes a **stretched muscle attached** to the Tendon to **relax** and signals its **opposing muscle to contract**. This action **protects** the stretched Muscle and Tendon from tearing.

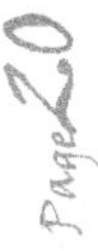

By **stretching** slowly during exercise, you avoid contracting the Muscle you are trying to **stretch**. As a **stretch** is held, your Muscles and Tendons **adapt to the new length**.

Flexibility: Ability to move a joint smoothly through a full range of motion.

Stretching: Primary method of improving flexibility.

Static or Passive stretching: Muscle is stretched naturally without force being applied.

Dynamic or Active stretching: Muscle is taken beyond its normal range of motion with help from a partner.

Time and Place

A **Stretch Workout** can be done **at any time** and **at any place** (e.g., first thing in the morning or last thing at night, while watching television, while waiting for someone, or while in a line), and during or after long periods of sitting, standing, or sleeping.

Factors That Influence Flexibility

- *Muscle temperature*. Warm muscles stretch more easily than cold muscles.

- *Physical activity*. Sedentary individuals are less flexible; active individuals tend to maintain or even increase flexibility.

- *Injury*. Injury can limit range of motion, but a good rehabilitation program can help regain all or part of a joint's flexibility.

- *Body composition*. Most muscular individuals have good flexibility because they have trained their muscles through a full range of motion. Overly bulky muscles may limit movement. Fat can also limit movement and flexibility.

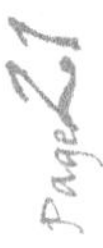

- *Age*. As a person ages, flexibility declines due more to inactivity than to the aging process itself. Flexibility can be maintained by doing stretching activities regularly.

- *Disease*. Diseases such as arthritis can make it uncomfortable or even painful to move joints. Arthritic individuals can improve their joint mobility through exercise.

- *Gender*. Females tend to have a slightly greater range of motion in most joints than males.

Benefits of Flexibility?

Flexibility offers the following benefits:

- **Increases** joint movement (mobility)

- **Improves circulation**, bringing nutrients to keep tissues healthy and transporting wastes out of the tissues

- **Improves performance** in some activities (e.g. golfing, dancing)

- **Improves posture and personal appearance**

- Assists in the cool-down phase of a workout

- **Reduces** the risk of low-back problems

- **Improves** coordination and balance, which helps maintain an Independent and Active lifestyle in the elderly

- Helps **reduce** excess stress by lowering anxiety and boosting feelings of self-confidence

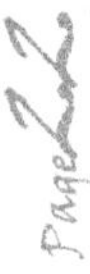

You can evaluate your posture by standing in front of a three-panel mirror of the kind often found in fitting rooms.

Why Have Good Posture?

- Good posture makes your bones align properly.

- Correct bone alignment allows for muscles, joints, and ligaments to work properly.

- With good posture, **internal organs are in the right position and can work more effectively** (allows for deep breathing and proper digestion).

- Good posture **lessens** the risk of lower-back pain.

- Good posture projects the body image that you are **Strong, Intelligent** and **Proud.**

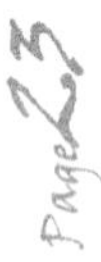

Signs of Poor Posture

- **Head aligned in front of center of gravity** (can cause headaches; dizziness; and neck, shoulder, and arm pain)

- **Too much outward curve in upper back** (can shorten breath by squeezing the lung area; can cause neck, shoulder, and arm pain)

- Too much inward curve in lower back (can cause low-back pain, painful menstruation)

- **Abdomen sticks out too far** (can cause <u>lordosis</u>, low-back pain, painful menstruation)

- **Knees extend backward too much** (can cause knee injury and lordosis)

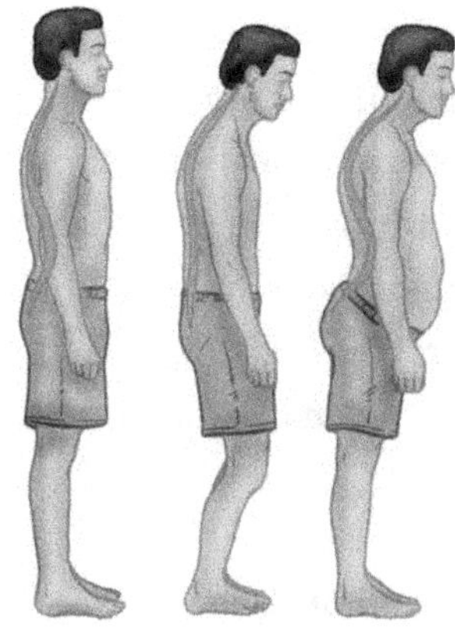

■ **Sit correctly:** Distribute your weight evenly on both hips, bend knees at a right angle, legs should not be crossed and feet should be flat on the floor, keep back straight and shoulders back.

■ **Stand correctly:** Hold **head up with chin in, ears should be in line with shoulders, shoulders should be back, chest forward, knees straight, stomach tucked in.**

(Picture: Left to right: good posture (pelvic tilt); poor posture (lordotic back, pelvis tilted too far forward; pelvis tilted too far back).

■ **Lift correctly:** Keep back straight and bend at knees and hips, keep feet in wide stance, lift object using leg muscles, moving in a steady motion.

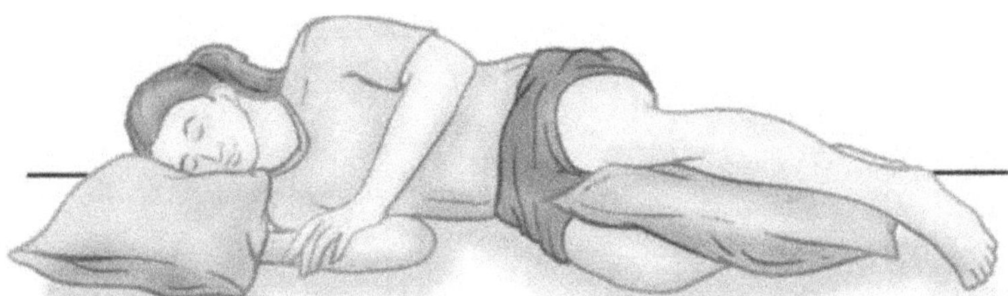

■ **Lie in bed correctly:** Lie on your side with your hips and knees slightly bent; put a flat pillow between your knee.

More than 80% of North Americans suffer back pain in their lifetime. **Low-back pain, both Acute and Chronic, centers on the Muscles *supporting* the Spine. Age and physical condition are the major factors associated with low-back pain,** along with the **trauma of lifting something in the wrong way** or **injuring yourself in an activity or sport.** Being overweight, poor posture, stress, and occupation (e.g., computer programmers and truck drivers) may contribute to the pain. There is also recent research indicating a link between smoking and lower-back pain.

The main cause of Lower-Back pain or discomfort stems from the Bodies inability to effectively communicate with itself ... whether it manifests in the form of NOT being able to transmit Energy or Electrical Signals ... it's the SAME results – PAIN and DISCOMFORT!

Acute: Rapid onset, severe symptoms, and short duration.

Chronic: Slow progression and long duration.

Preventing Low-Back Pain

To prevent low-back pain:

- Exercise regularly to improve the **strength** of your Back and Abdominal Muscles.

- Maintain **correct posture** in sitting and **standing**, especially while studying and working on a computer.

- **Warm up before engaging in physical activity.**

- Keep the spine **straight up** and **down** when **lifting** an object. **Do not bend over.** Use the muscles of your Legs and Hips to lift.

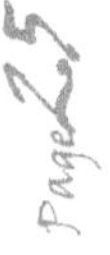

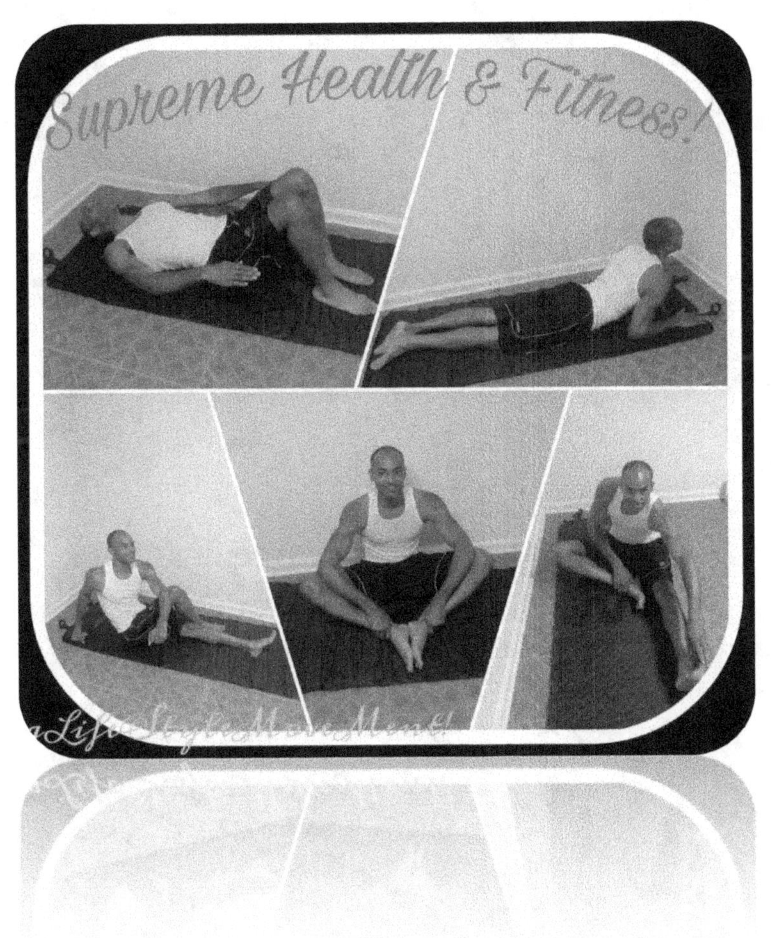
Supreme Health & Fitness!

*****

Exercises for Lower-Back Pain Relief

*****

The following Activities will help to Stretch and Strengthen your lower-back to Improve and Increase Your Energy Flow ... All the following Activities are to be performed SLOWLY as to prevent further or new injury:

Activity 1: Get Up to Life Supreme Curl-up

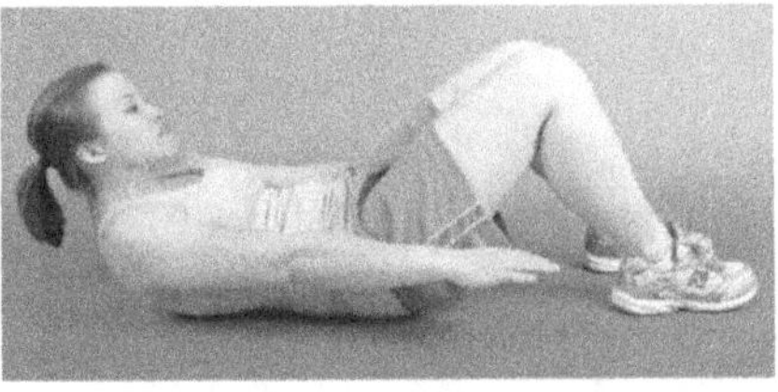

This activity is designed to offer a comfortable stretch of your entire Spine/Back, with particular focus on your Lumbar region ... with MINIMAL dis-comfort, pain or

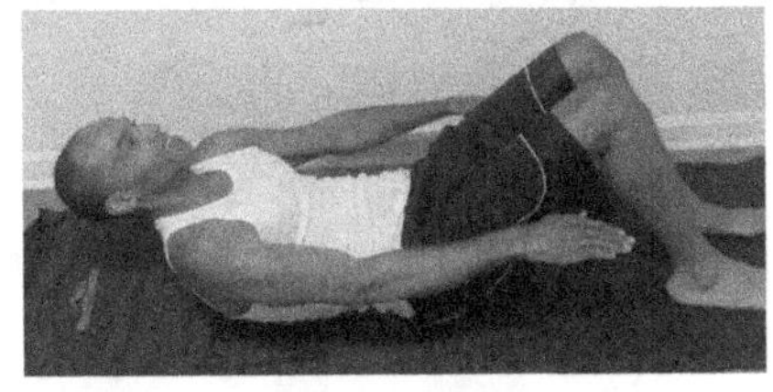

further injury ... Directions: Lay flat on your back, knees bent at comfortable 45* angle (where your feet lay flat) and hands at side. Slowly raise your Shoulders (keep head straight and lifting the shoulders only) approximately 4-6 inches off the ground. Hold for 10-15 seconds - Slowly Lower, Relax and Repeat - 10-reps

*****

Activity 2: Twist the Pain Away Supreme Elbow to Knee Stretch

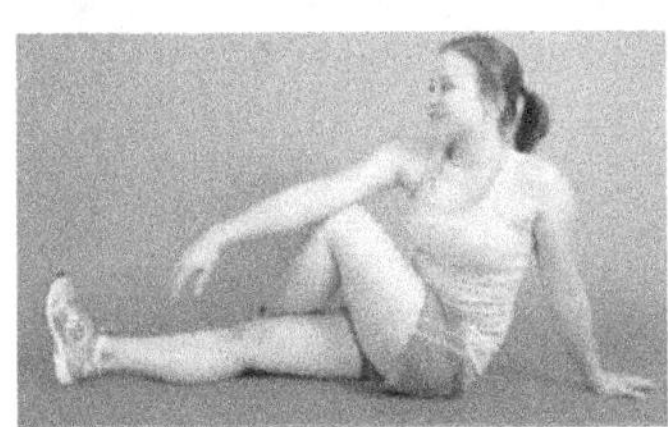

This activity is designed to help Strengthen and simultaneously offer Relief to Your Lumbar region. This activity helps to reinvigorate the Lumbar region by helping to increase the Blood, Energy and Electrical flow to Growth, Development and Relief.

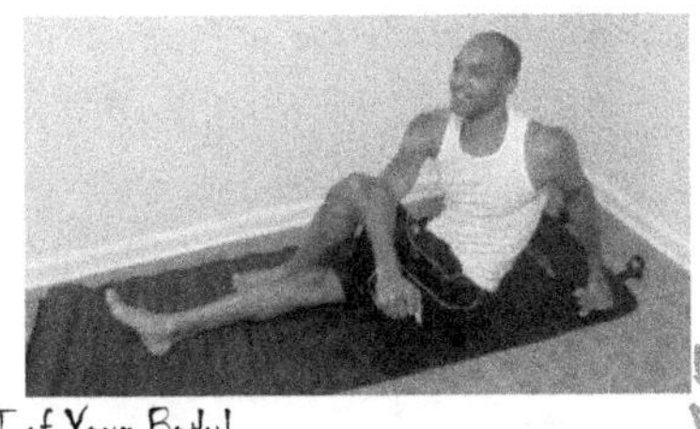

Envision the Twisting Motion squeezing all the Tension and Pain OUT of Your Body!

*****

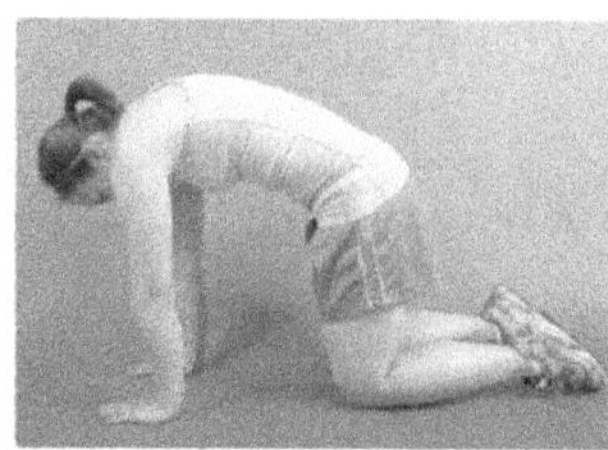

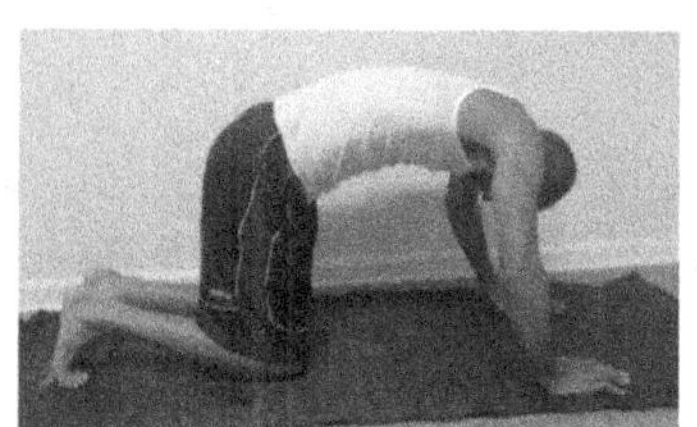

Activity 3: Supreme Camel & Cat Stretch

These are Fun and very Effective Activities that you can Immediately feel in an almost instant sensation of Relief!

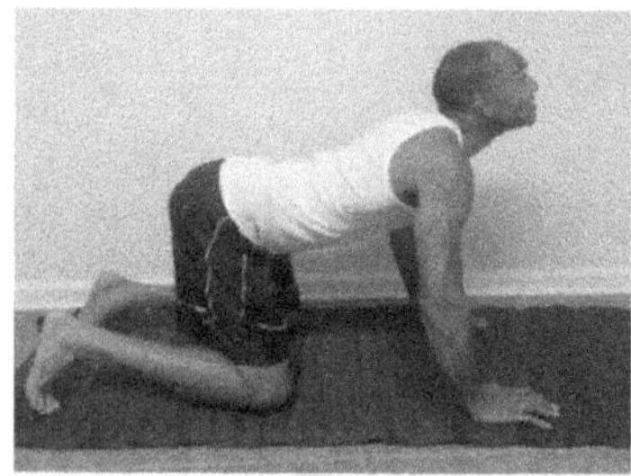

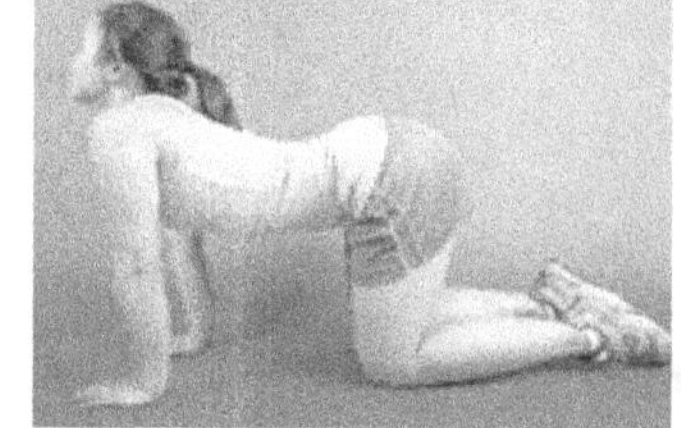

While performing these Activities You can Feel the Restoration of the Flow of Life Energy thru Your Body!
You can perform these Activities as precautionary measures or for relief as needed.
These rea Great Activities to Begin and End Your day with!

*****

Activity 4: Get the Pain off me Supreme Chest Lift:

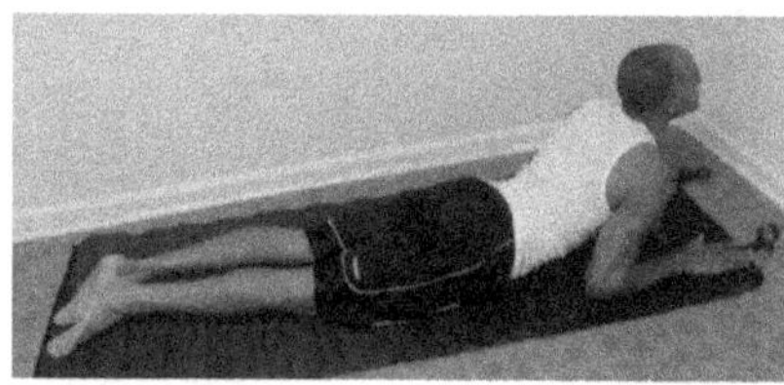

This is a Great Activity to release the Pressure that can build-up in the Lumbar region from lack of Energy Flow ... The 1st sign of an Energy

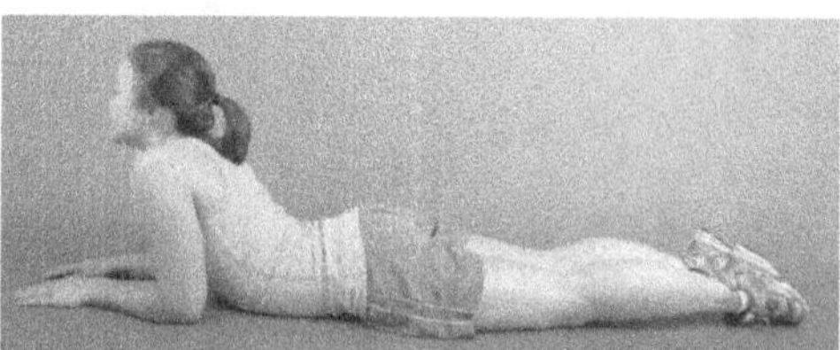

blockage is Pain, Tension or Discomfort. As you are performing this Activity, Envision You Lifting and Pushing the Pain right OUT of Your Back!

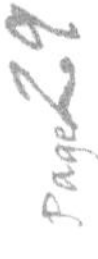

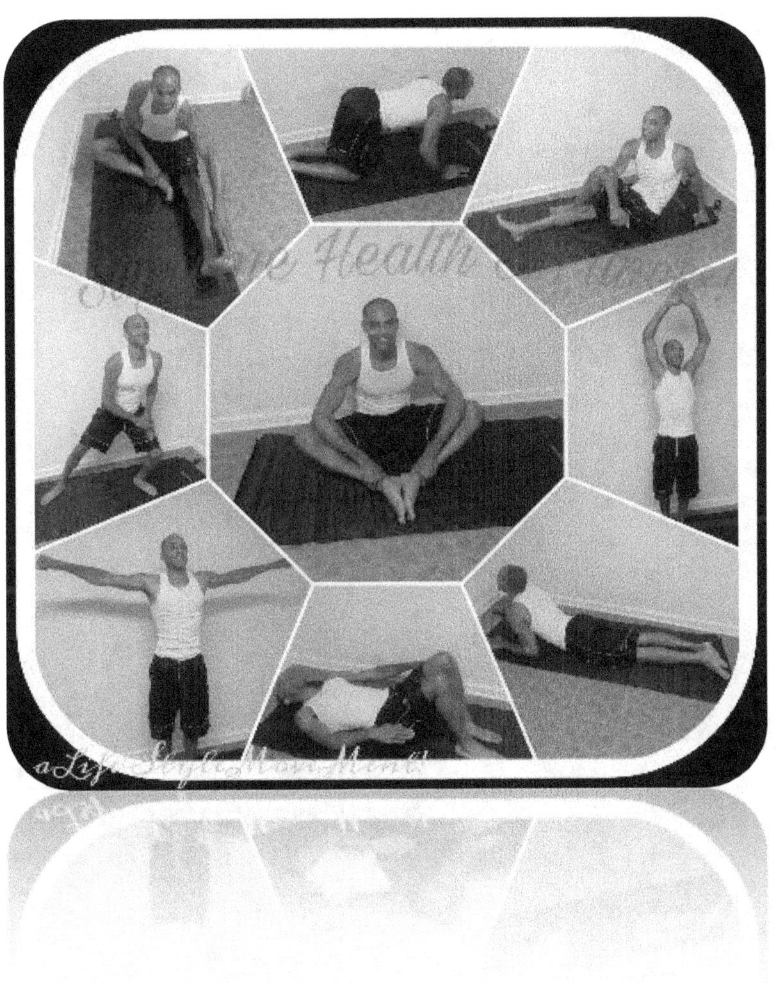

Creating a Flexibility Program

*****

The adage **"use it or lose it"** applies especially to **flexibility**. Joint flexibility **decreases** with aging; however, it can be **improved** through exercises.

Each **muscle–tendon** group joint is different; we need to do exercises **specific** for each Joint to maintain or improve its range of motion. There is no one specific test of overall flexibility, so you should plan a program of stretching exercises that involves most of your joints (e.g., shoulder, chest, neck, trunk, lower back, hips, and posterior and anterior legs).

Precautions involving stretching include:

- Do not stretch swollen or painful joints without a healthcare professional's advice.

- Do not stretch a surgically repaired joint without a healthcare professional's advice.

- Avoid potentially harmful stretching exercises.

The Supreme Health & Fitness F.I.T.T. Formula for Flexibility

The goal of our Flexibility program - develop & increase the **range of motion** in all major joints.

F = Frequency: Performing flexibility activities **2 to 3 days per week** is effective, but greater gains in **joint range of motion** can be obtained with **daily flexibility activities**.

I = Intensity: **Stretch** to the point of **mild** discomfort or tightness.

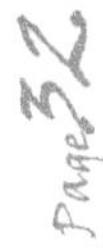

T = Time: Holding a stretch for **10–30 seconds** at the **point of tightness** or slight discomfort **enhances joint range of motion**. Holding it longer offers no additional benefit except in older persons who may **gain greater improvements** in **range of motion** with a **30- to 60-second stretch.**

Repetitions of 2-4 times for each flexibility activity is effective. The Goal is to gain **60 seconds of total stretching time per flexibility exercise** (e.g., 60 seconds of stretch time can be met by two 30-second stretches or four 15-second stretches).

Completing a daily set of flexibility activities can be completed within **10 minutes.**

When to stretch? Do not stretch to warm up. Flexibility activities are most effective when the Muscles are **warmed through light-to-moderate cardiorespiratory** or **muscular endurance exercise** or through **external-moist heat packs or hot baths**. You will gain the most flexibility by **stretching after your cardiorespiratory** or **resistance exercise is completed.**

 Flexibility exercise can be done alone—not involving other types of exercise.

T = Types of Stretching: Stretching techniques include **Static** stretches, **Dynamic** stretches, **Ballistic** stretches, and **PNF** (Proprioceptive Neuromuscular Facilitation).

Static Stretching: Static stretching is the **most common** and **practical** type of stretching. It is effective, causes less pain, and usually is easier to do. Perform a **static stretch** by **slowly** and **gently** stretching the muscle to the **point of tightness** and holding that position for **10–30 seconds.**

Dynamic Stretching: Dynamic or **slow-movement stretching** involves a gradual transition from one body position to another and a progressive **increase** in **reach** and **range of motion** as the movement is repeated several times. This involves **moving a Joint through its full range of motion with little resistance.** The movement can be through the range of motion used in a specific exercise or sport.

Ballistic Stretching: Ballistic stretching uses bouncing, repetitive movements to force a stretch past the normal range of motion. When properly performed, it is as effective as static stretching and may be considered for those engaged in ballistic movements (e.g., basketball).

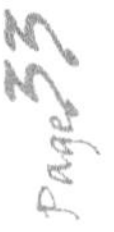

PLEASE: CONSULT YOUR HEALTH CARE PROVIDER BEFORE YOU BEGIN THIS OR ANY EXERCISE ACTIVITY!!

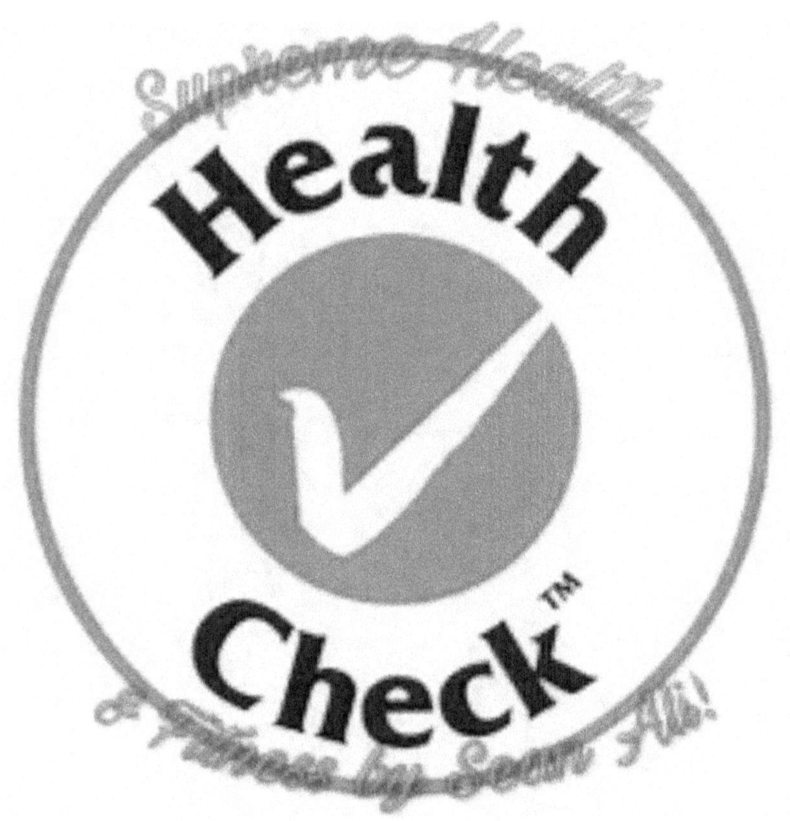

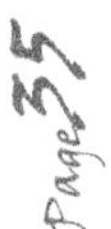

Easy At-Home (or on-the-go) Stretching Activities:

*****

Stretching Increases Blood Flow and significantly Improves our Ability to Move and the Duration. Proper Blood Flow to our Brain is Key to Over-All physical and mentally Health and Wellness.

These EASY Activities Start at the TOP — Increasing Energy to our Brain, and then working the way down, following our natural path of Blood Circulation.

REMEMBER ... Stretching is FUN and EASY... Stretching is designed to LOOSEN your Muscular Structures, IMPROVE your Life Energy Circulation, RELAX your Mind and STIMULATE YOU INTO MOTION!!!!

In some pictures, the example of the Activities are Outside. I wanted to demonstrate the Importance and Ease of performing as many Activities as possible OUTSIDE. And if permissible, with as less clothing as needed (especially NO SHOES!) to Create the CONNECTIVE environment between You, Mother Earth, Oxygen and The CREATOR!!!!

PLEASE ... HAVE FUN, ENJOY AND BE ALIVE!!!

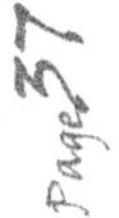

*Upper Body Activities ... Shoulders * Chest * Upper Back * Abdominals!

Activity 1: Get the Blood Flowing Supreme Neck Stretching

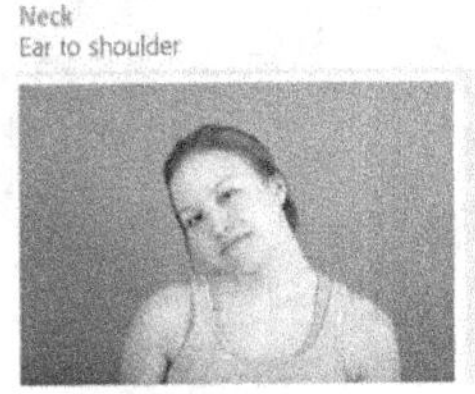

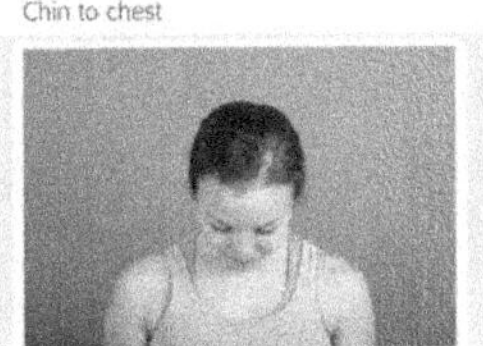

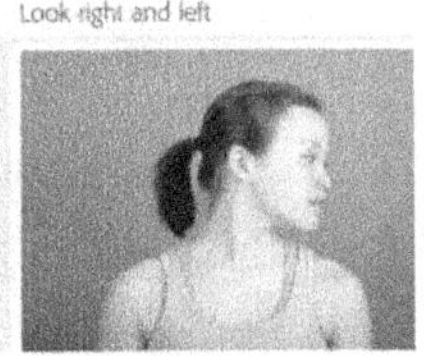

****

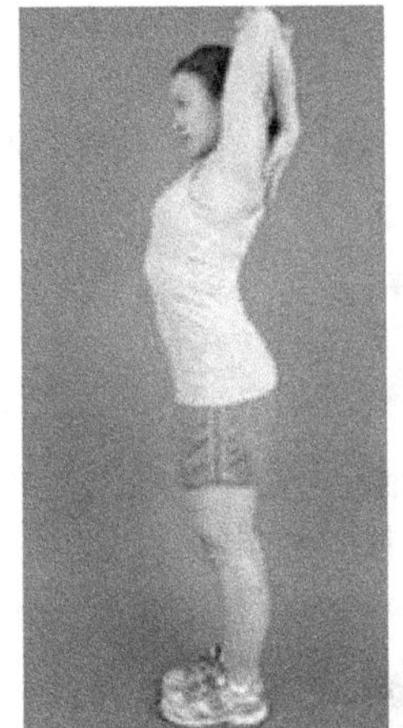

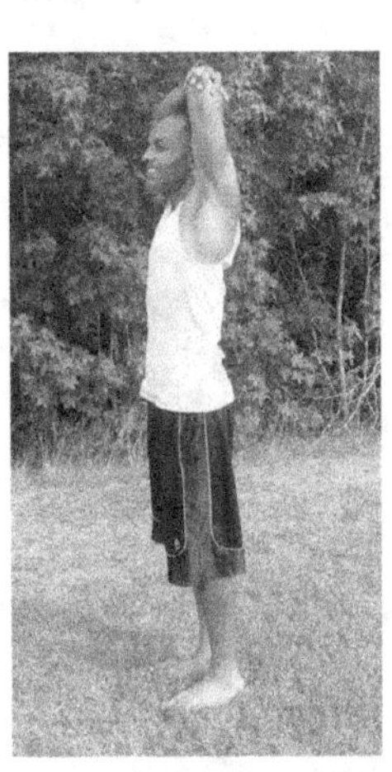

Activity 2: Self Congratulating Supreme Back Stretch!

Slowly raise Arm to postion Hand COMFORTABLY on Shoulder Blade...Use the FIIT Guides .. 10-30 secs. 2-4-reps

*****

Activity 3: Reaching for My Goals Supreme Stretch-Ups!

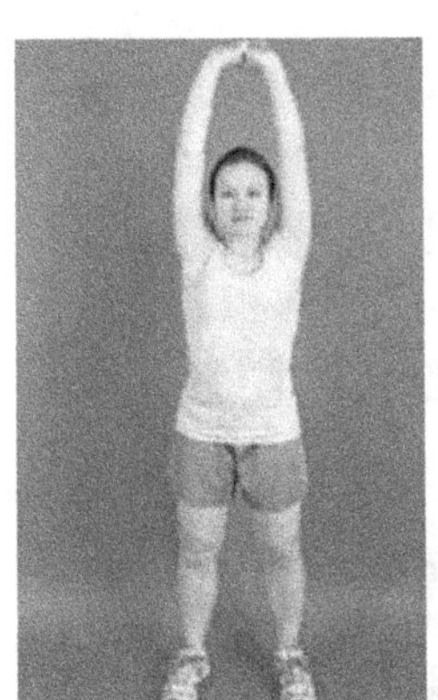

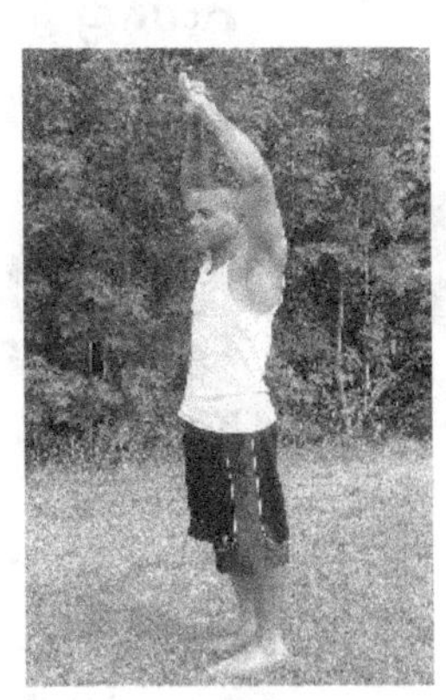

Picture Your Goals up above your Head...SLOWLY raise both arms, joining Hands over-head. Picture Grabbing Your Goals ... Hold for 10-30 secs ... SLOWLY lower your Arms with Your Goals In them...4-reps = 4 Goals!

Activity 4: Winding the Heart Supreme Slow Arm Roll!

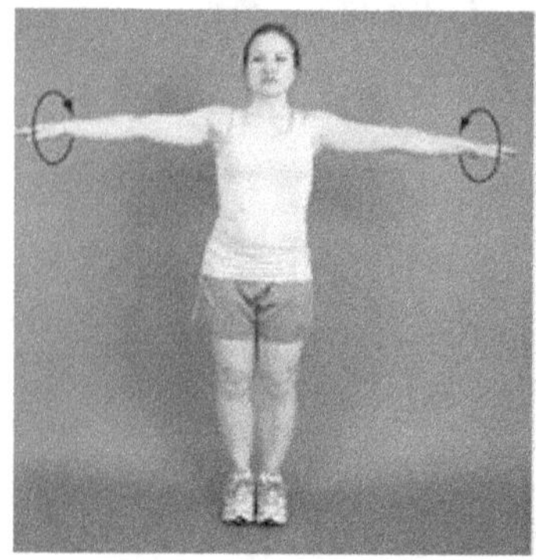

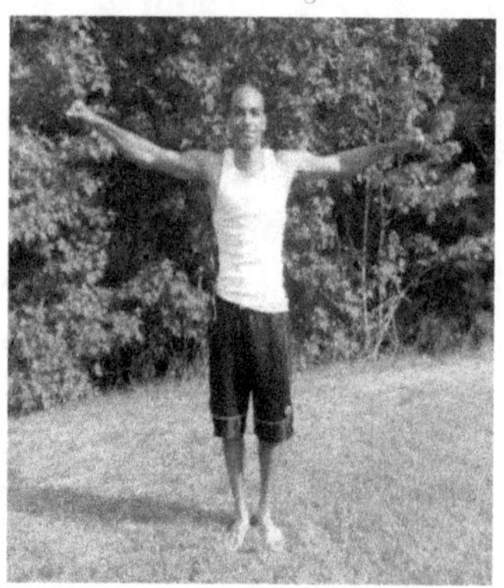

In this Activity, as you SLOWLY extend your Arms. picture them being CONNECTED to Your Heart .. As you Slowly rotate them for 10-30 seconds .. Picture Your Heart being Wound-Up with Life Energy!

Activity 5: Supreme Shoulder Roll the Tension AWAY!

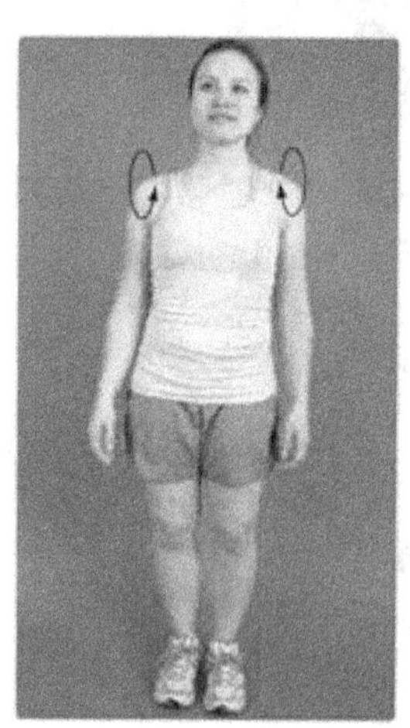

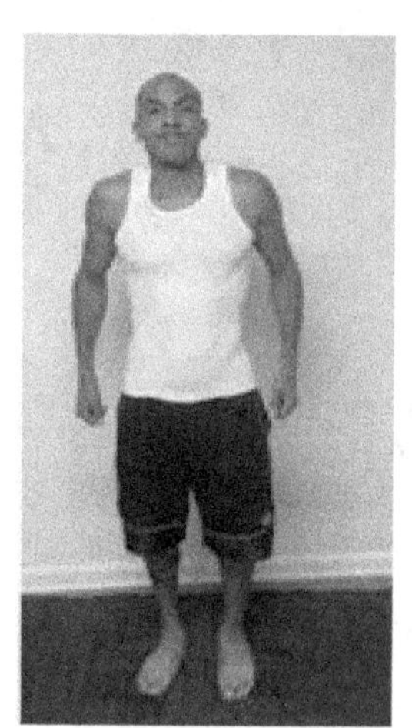

As you are performing this Activity, Imagine that with each Shoulder Roll you can SEE the Tension, Worries and Pain LEAVE Your Body ... Remember, Stretching is done at a SLOW pace!

Perform the Rolls for 10-30 secs .. for 4-reps

*****

Activity 6: Tension and Stress Reliever Supreme Wall Press!

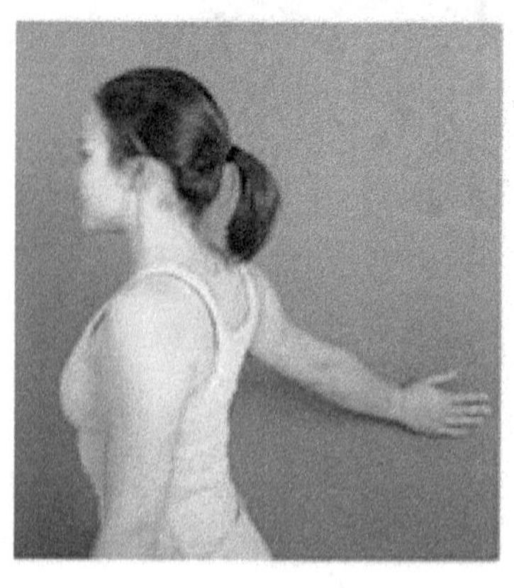

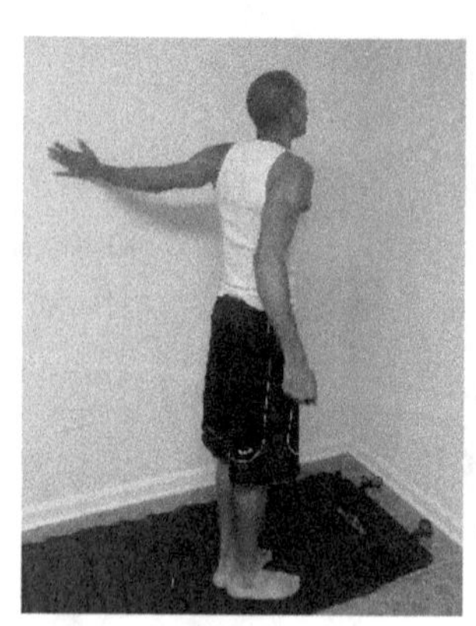

As you slow place each arm on the wall, Palms facing away from you, you slowly apply pressure until you can feel the tension in your Shoulders and Chest. As you are performing this Activity, picture the wall as Your source of Tension, Stress or Pain ... For the count of 5-10 seconds ... SEE YOURSELF PUSHING THEM AWAY!!!! ... 10-30 secs .. 4-reps

Activity 7: Getting the Monkey off your Back Supreme Shoulder Stretch

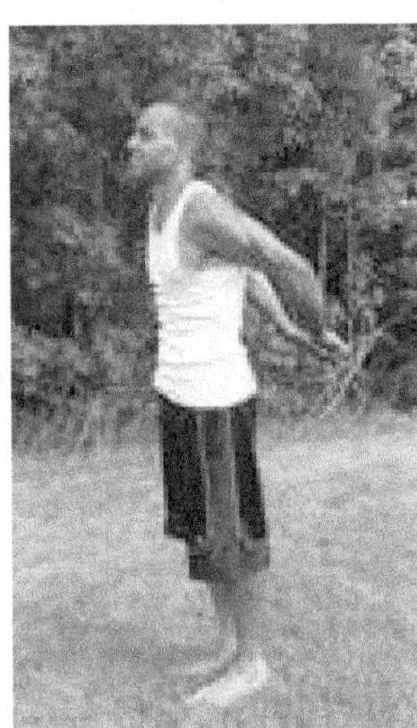

As You're performing this Activity- Picture any Tension or Stress from Your Shoulders to Your Lumbar region LEAVING Your Body as you extend Your Arms backwards — away from Your Body.

Perform for 10-30 secs .. 4-reps

*****

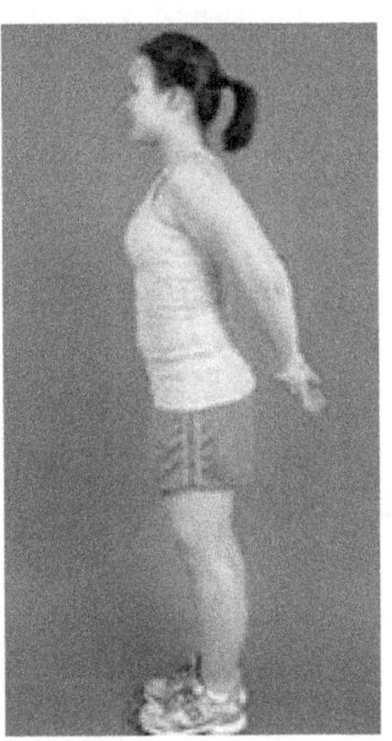

*Lower Body Activities ... Quads * Thighs * Hips

Activity 1: Supreme Butterfly

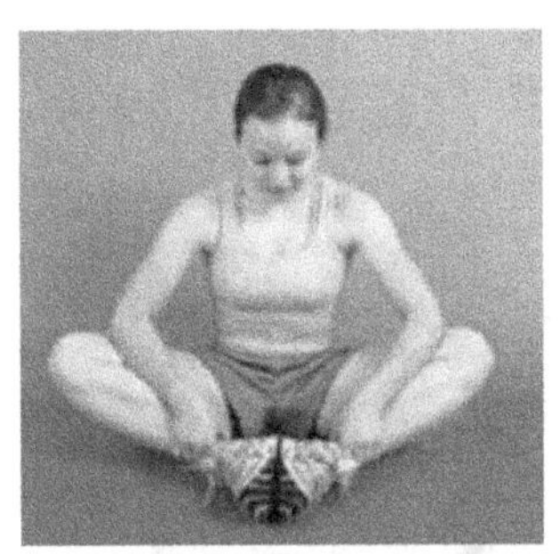

This is a Fun Activity that takes you back to your childhood!

As You sit Comfortably on the floor, with Bottom of Feet placed together, place your Elbows on your Knees ... SLOWLY push down on Your Knees – until You reach the point of Discomfort .. Hold 10-30 secs .. Relax ... Repeat 4-reps

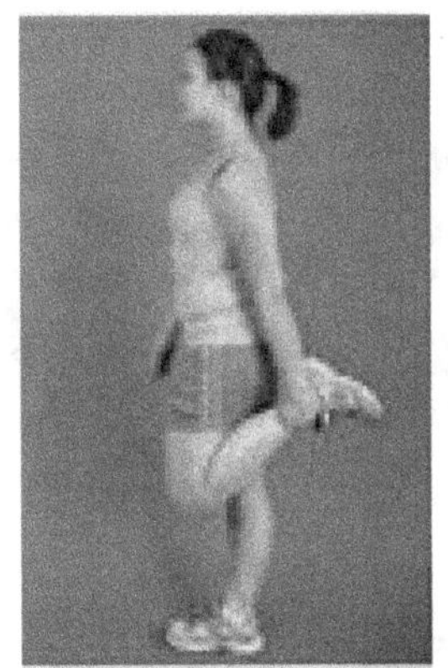

*****

Activity 2: Supreme Standing Knee-to-Buttocks

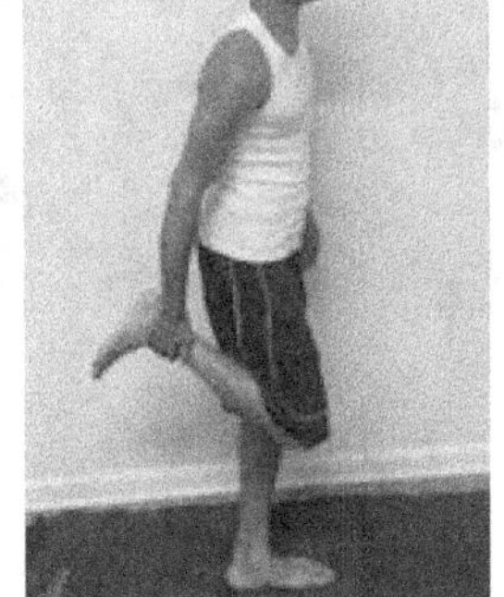

(Please – If You Have ANY Prior Knee PAIN Or INJURY – CONTACT YOUR HEALTH CARE PROVIDER)

*****

Activity 3: Dodging Stress Supreme Side Lunge

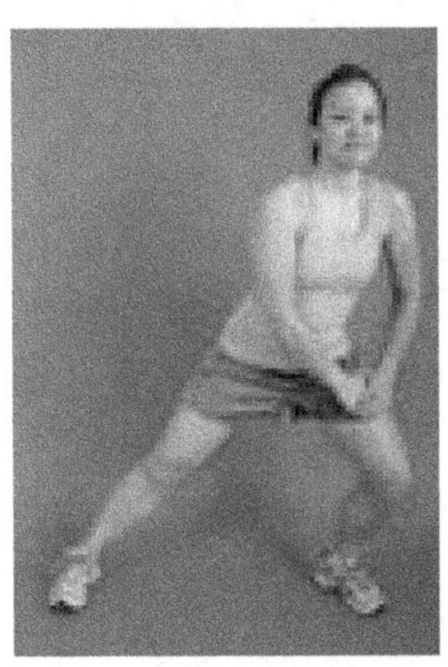

This world is full of Stressors and "Haters" ... as You perform this Activity, Picture that Your DODGING all the Stress and Hate as you SLOWLY extend one Leg while Balancing and shifting Your weight on the Leg NOT extended ... Hold 10-30 seconds ... Relax ... Switch Legs ... And DODGE MORE STRESS TO A MORE FLEXIBLE YOU!!

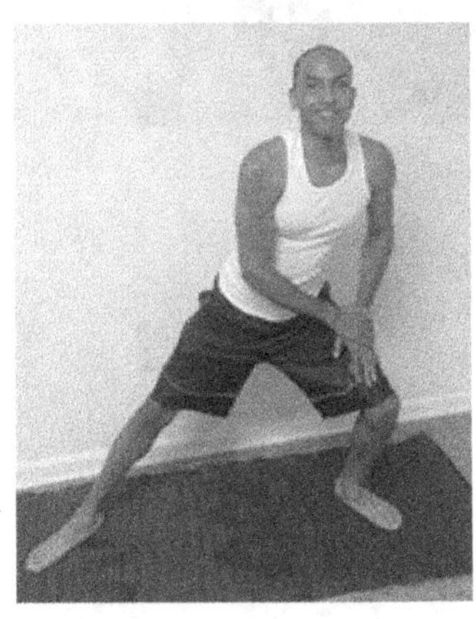

*****

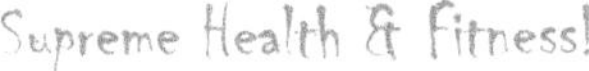

*Lower Body ... Hamstrings * Groin * Lower-Back

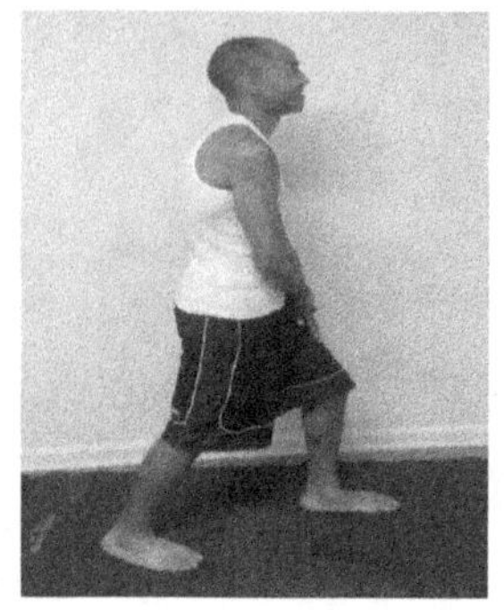

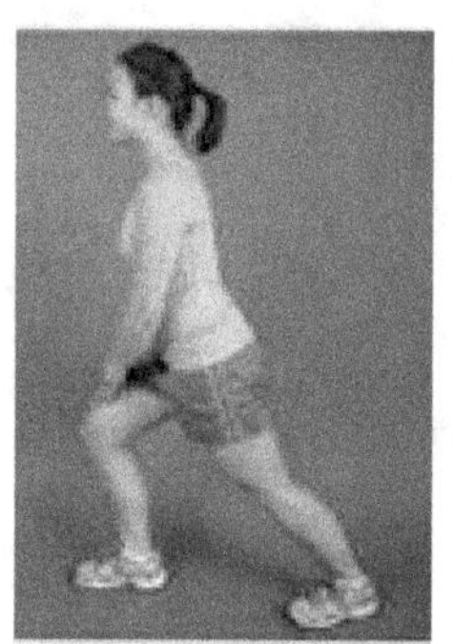

Activity 4: Standing Firm Supreme Forward Standing Lunge

As you perform this Activity, imagine that you are Standing Firm against any Stress, Discomfort, Dis-ease or Pain that can come your Way ... Hold the position for 10-30 secs ... alternating Legs ... 4-reps!

*****

Activity 5: The Fly-Away from Stress Supreme Super-Man Stretch!

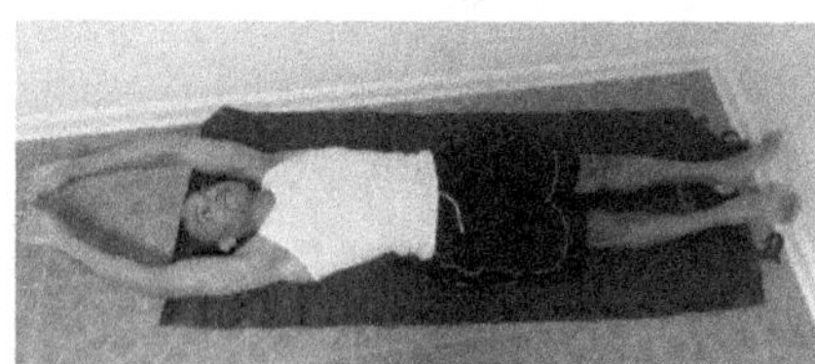

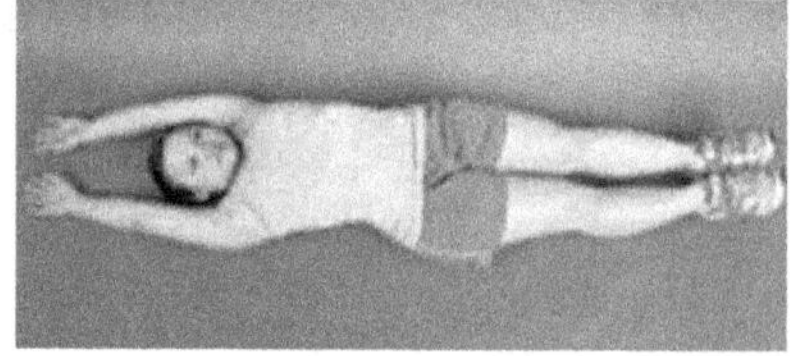

This is one of my Favorite Stretching Activities. As you are performing this Activity ... Imagine that you are Flying AWAY from any Stress, Pain or Discomfort ... FEEL YOUR BODY FILLING WITH LIFE ENERGY!

*****

Activity 5: Supreme Hamstring Stretch!

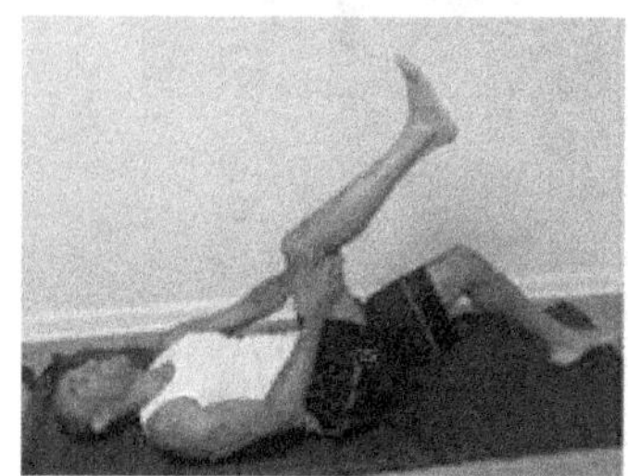

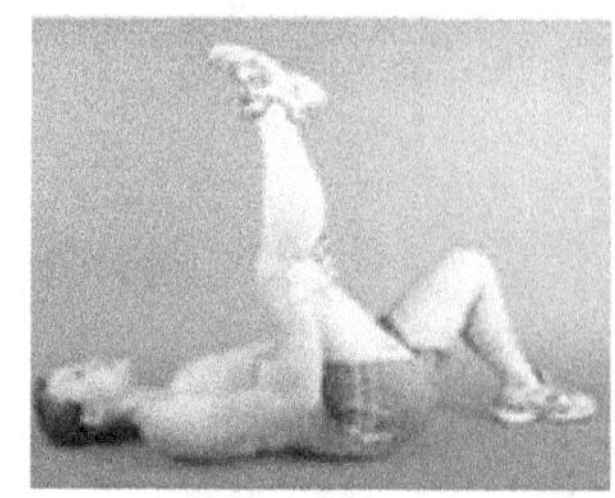

This Activity is designed to open-up the Flow of Energy to Your Legs. Most pain occurs as a Signal that we are lacking in Electrical Flow, which Stretching helps Restore!

*****

Activity 6: Supreme Knee-to-Chest Stretch

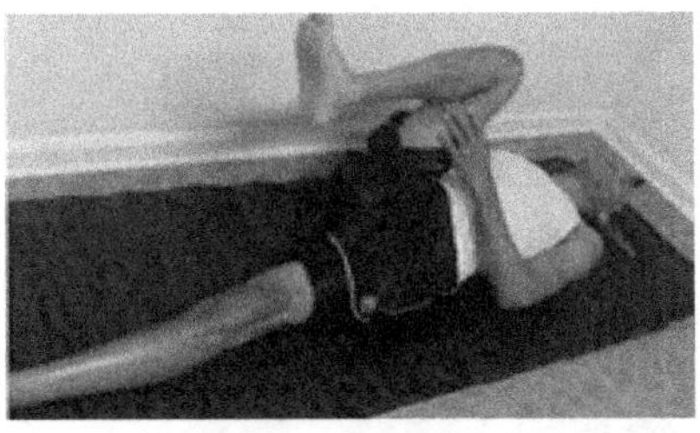

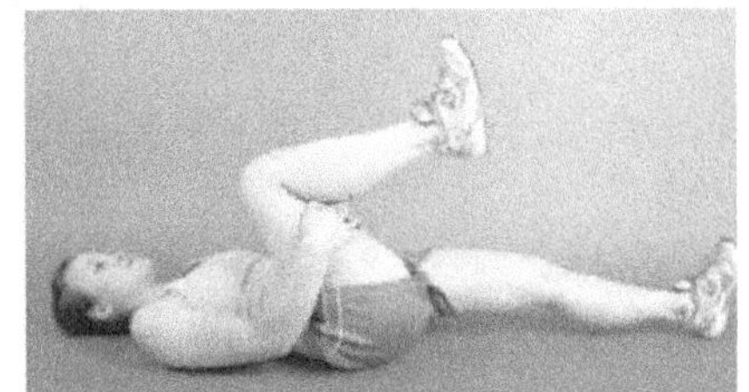

As you are performing this stretch, you can Feel the Tension, Discomfort or Pain LEAVE Your Body and the Muscles and Tissues RELAX!

That Good Feeling is the Restoration of Your Flow of Life Energy!

As you SLOWLY Stretch and hold the position for 5-10 seconds before SLOWLY Relaxing ... Concentrate on PEACE and Visualizing YourSelf Enjoying Abundant Life!!!

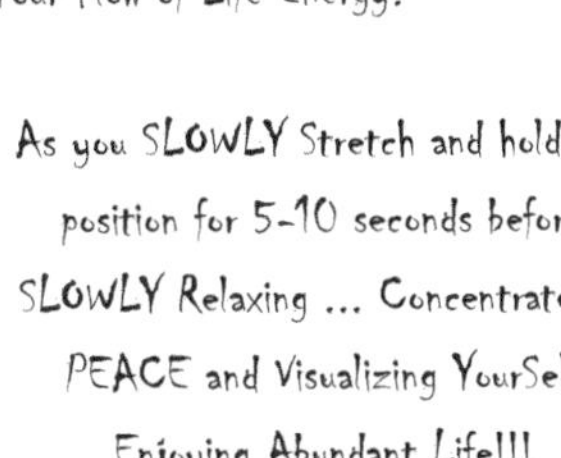

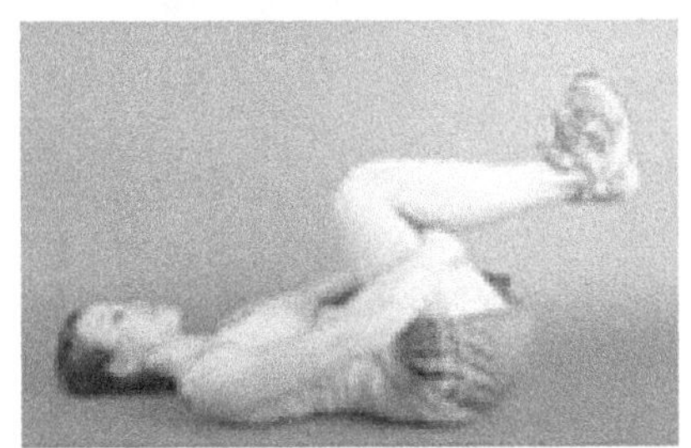

*****

Activity 7: Over-Coming Stress Supreme Hurdler

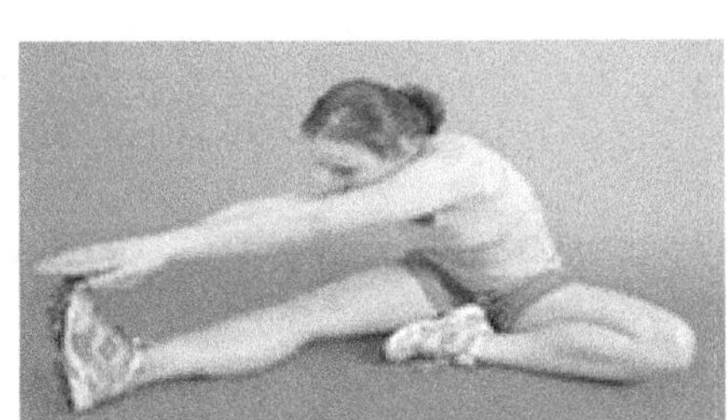

This is referred to as the Herdle Stretch because you mimic the Action of a Hurdler ... So as you perform this Activity Envision YourSelf Hurdling OVER All Your Stress and Pain!!

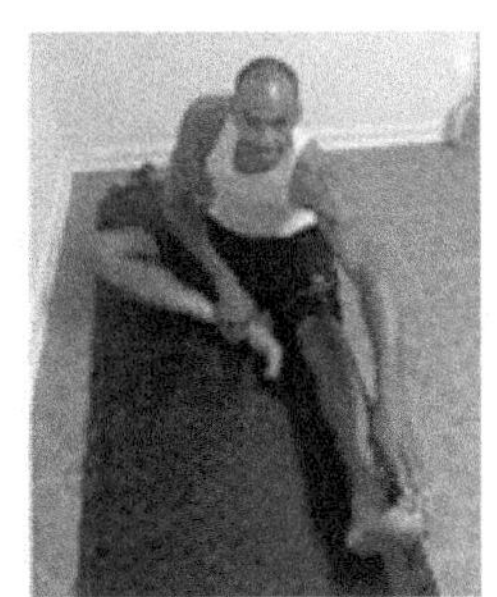

Activity 8: Pushing Stress AWAY Supreme Calf Stretch

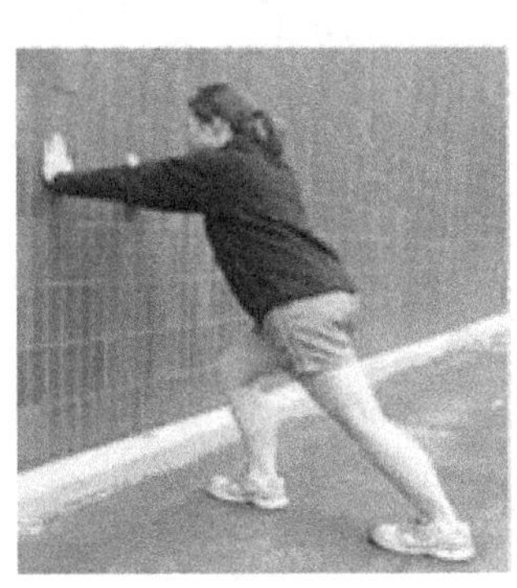

While You are performing this Activity, Envision YourSelf HOLDING BACK and PUSHING AWAY All Your Stress, Tension and Pain ... Pushing them Right OUT of Your Body and LIFE!

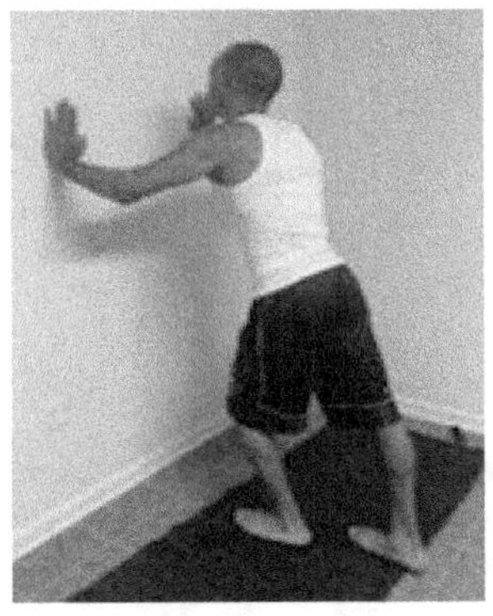

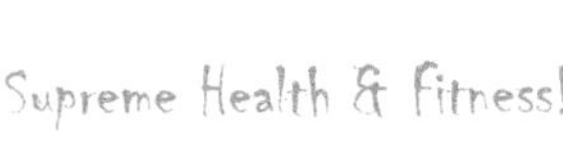

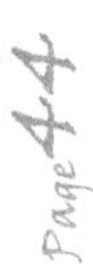

• Avoid **ballistic stretching** – like, bending forcefully to touch your toes with your knees straight and bouncing while you reach. Ballistic stretching may do more harm than good, because the muscles may shorten reflexively. This stretching is not recommended for most people.

Informal Stretching

Stretching can be done virtually anywhere. When you need a quick break, want a short stress reliever (during a test, for instance), or sense discomfort in a muscle group during the day, use stretching as a means to relieve the pain. In addition, these activities can be fun if you choose to do them with a friend, while listening to music or watching television, or during your own time. Here is an example of a routine you can do anywhere, anytime:

- Clasp your hands together and stretch out in front of you.

- In the same position, stretch your hands over your head.

- While standing or sitting, lean right.

- While standing or sitting, lean left.

- Clasp your hands behind your back and open up your chest area.

- Stretch your wrists by bending your wrists back, then down, then in a circle.

- Lift your shoulders up to your ears, then down and back. Do that five times.

- Take your right hand and put it on your left shoulder. With your left hand, gently push your right elbow, pushing your right hand past your shoulder and stretching the back of your right arm.

- Stretch your left arm in the same manner.

- Put your hands flat on your desk, palms down, and push your chair out, stretching your back.

- Feel free to add more stretches for variety and to avoid boredom!

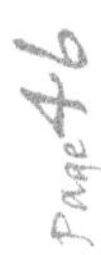

Think about the activities you do and the postures you assume each day. Are there ways you can **Improve** your **Flexibility** and **Posture** just by changing the way you do these activities?

When you are either *sitting* or *standing*, are you:

■ Arching your back?

■ Rounding your shoulders?

■ Letting your head slump forward?

When you are *lying* down, are you:

■ Tilting your pelvis down?

■ Arching your back?

While lying on your back, you should have just enough room between the small of your back and the floor to slide a computer mouse under there. You know your posture is bad if your back is touching the floor (squishing the mouse) or arching (the mouse could do jumping jacks).

Consciously **change what you do during each *activity* or *posture*. For instance:**

■ While sitting, keep your back straight, lean slightly forward, and use a footrest to keep your knees higher than your hips.

■ While standing, use a footrest to raise one leg to help you keep your back straight.

■ When lifting, bend at the knees, not at the waist, lift slowly, and push with your legs. Do not twist.

■ Do one different stretching activity each morning, at noon, and each evening before going to bed.

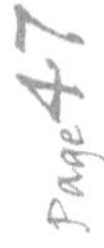

Remember that when performing ANY Stretching exercise, you are placing additional Stress on your Joints, Ligaments, Tendons and Muscles….ALL of which have a high degree of potential for INJURY!!!

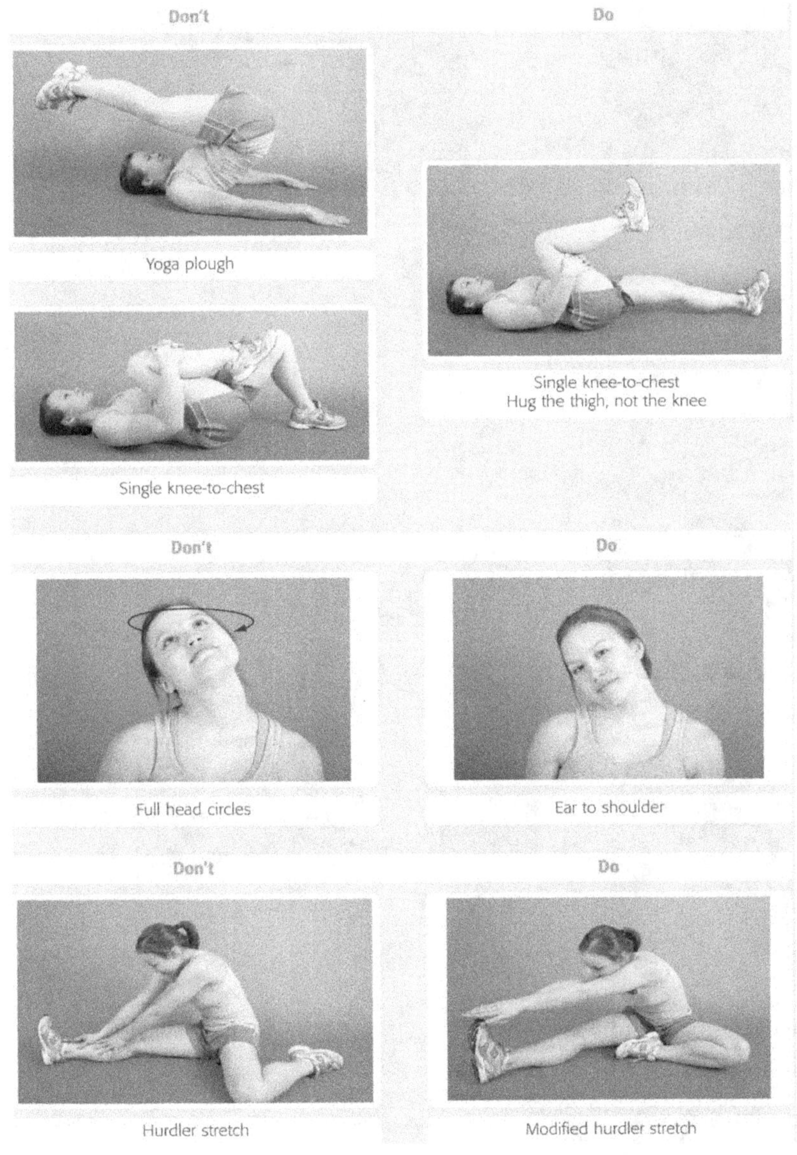

Don't

Do

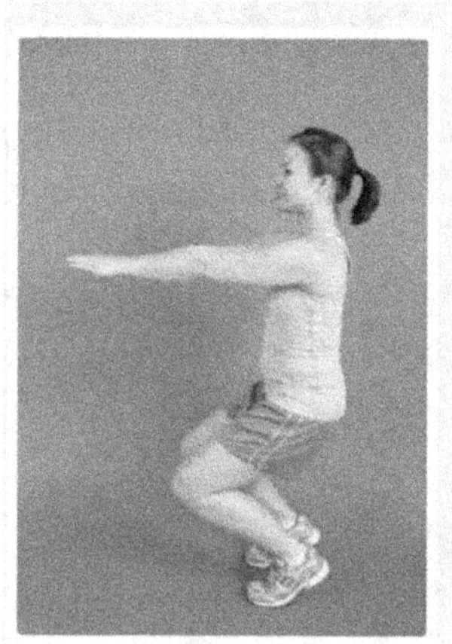

Full squat

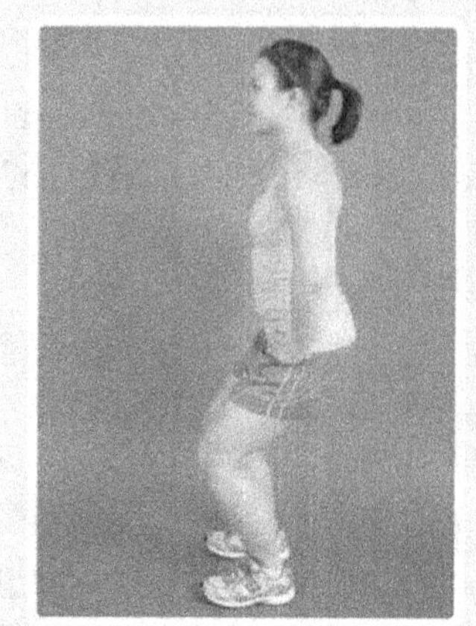

Half-knee bend

Don't

Do

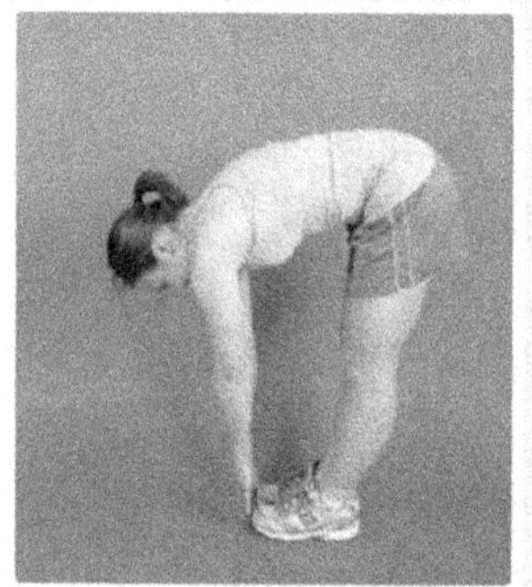

Standing toe touch

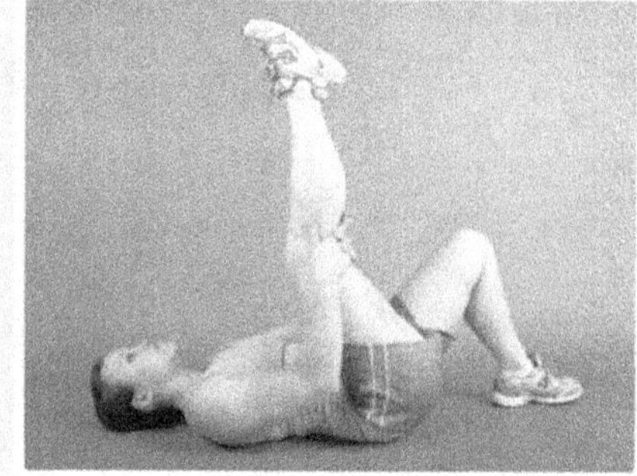

Lying hamstring stretch

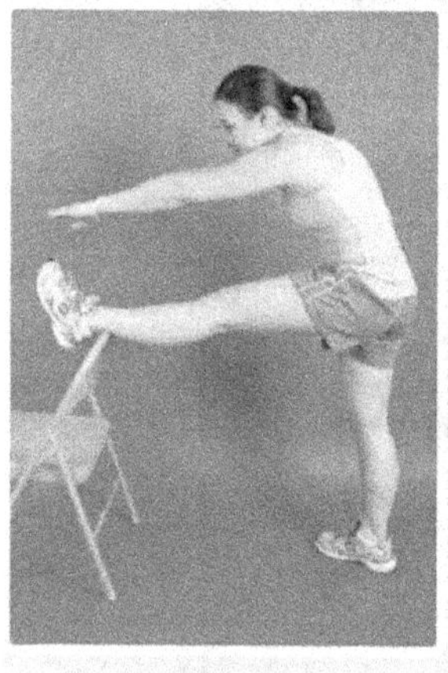

Ballet bar leg stretch

Don't

Do

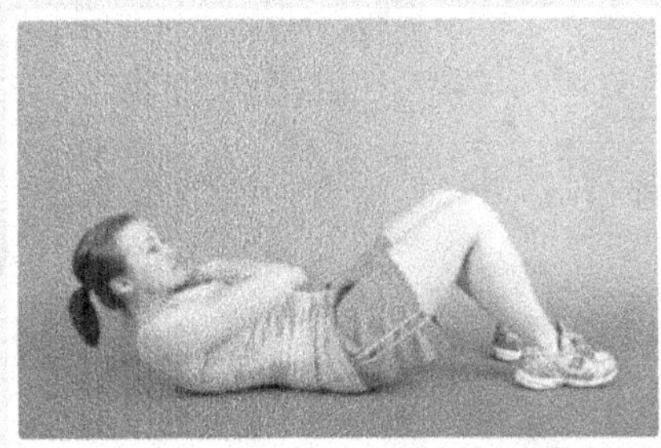

Straight-leg sit-ups with hands behind head

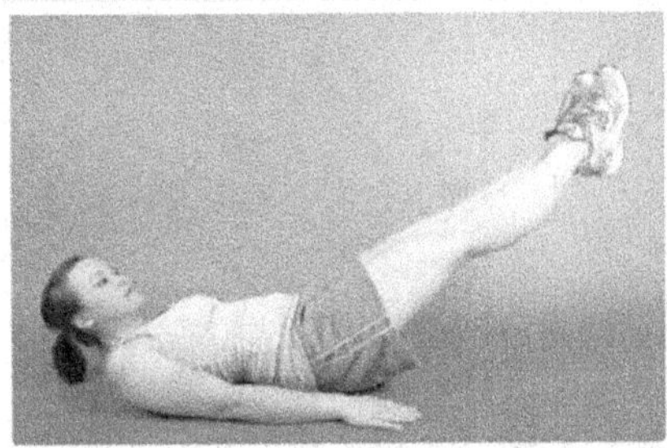

Bent-knee abdominal curls

Double-leg lifts

*****

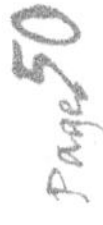

American Academy of Orthopedic Surgeons: *http://aaos.org*

MedlinePlus: *http://www.nlm.nih.gov/medlineplus*

National Institute on Aging: *http://www.nia.nih.gov*

Physician and Sports Medicine: *http://www.physsportsmed.org*

*References and Suggested Readings

———. Stretching during warm-up: Do we have enough evidence? *Journal of Physical Education, Recreation and Dance* 2000; 70:271–277.

American College of Sports Medicine. Quantity and Quality of Exercise for Developing and Maintaining Cardiorespiratory, Musculoskeletal, and Neuromotor Fitness in Apparently Healthy Adults: Guidance for Prescribing Exercise. *Medicine and Science in Sports and Exercise.* DOI: 10.1249/MSS.0b0138213fefb

Canham-Chervak M., et al. Does stretching before exercise prevent lower-limb injury? *Clinical Journal of Sport Medicine* 2000; 10:216.

Garber, C. E., et al. Quantity and quality of exercise for developing and maintaining cardiorespiratory, musculoskeletal, and neuromotor fitness in apparently healthy adults: Guidance for prescribing exercise. *Medicine and Science in Sports and Exercise* 2011; 43(7): 1334–1359.

Gleim G. W. and McHugh M. P. Flexibility and its effect on sports injury and performance. *Sports Medicine* 1997; 24:289–299.

Hodges P. and Jull G. Does strengthening the abdominal muscles prevent low-back pain? *Journal of Rheumatology* 2000; 27:2286–2288.

Knudson D. Stretching: From science to practice. *Journal of Physical Education, Recreation and Dance* 1998; 69:38–42.

Patel A. T. and Ogle A. A. Diagnosis and management of acute low back pain. *American Family Physician* 2000; 61:1779–1786.

Shrier I. and Gossal K. Myths and truths of stretching. *Physician and Sports Medicine* 2000; 28:57–63.

Shrier I. Stretching before exercise: An evidence-based approach. *British Journal of Sports Medicine* 2000; 34:324–325.

U.S. DHHS. *2008 Physical Activity Guidelines for Americans.* www.health.gov/paguidelines

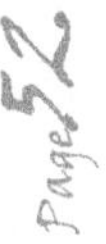

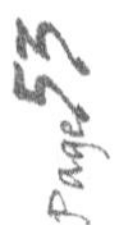

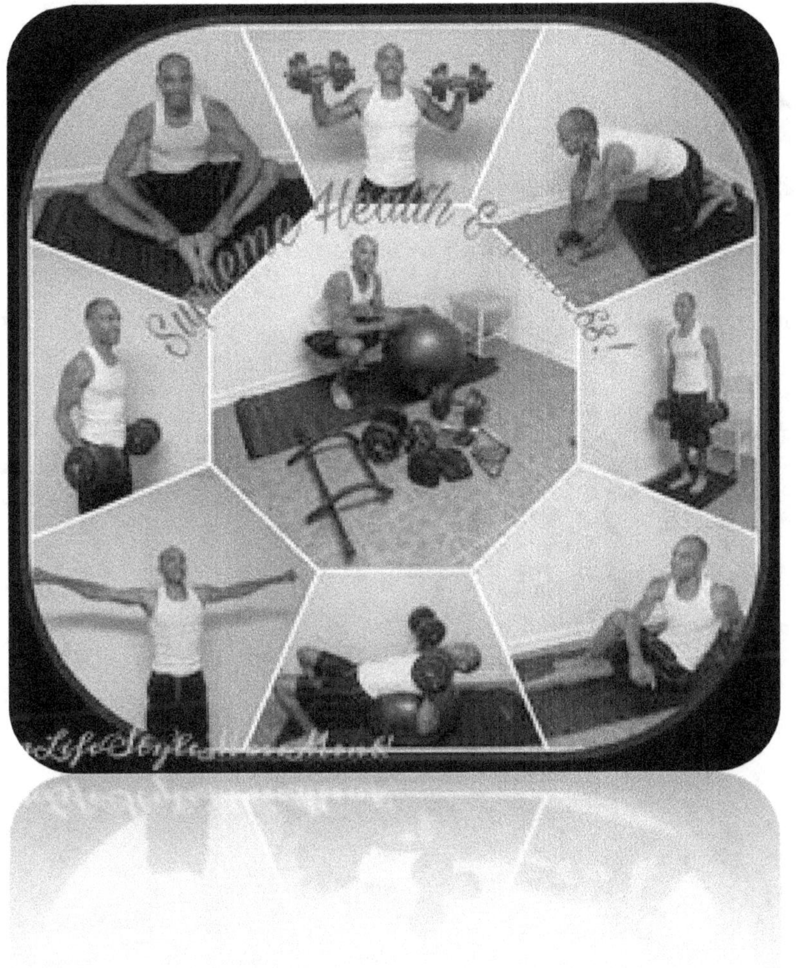

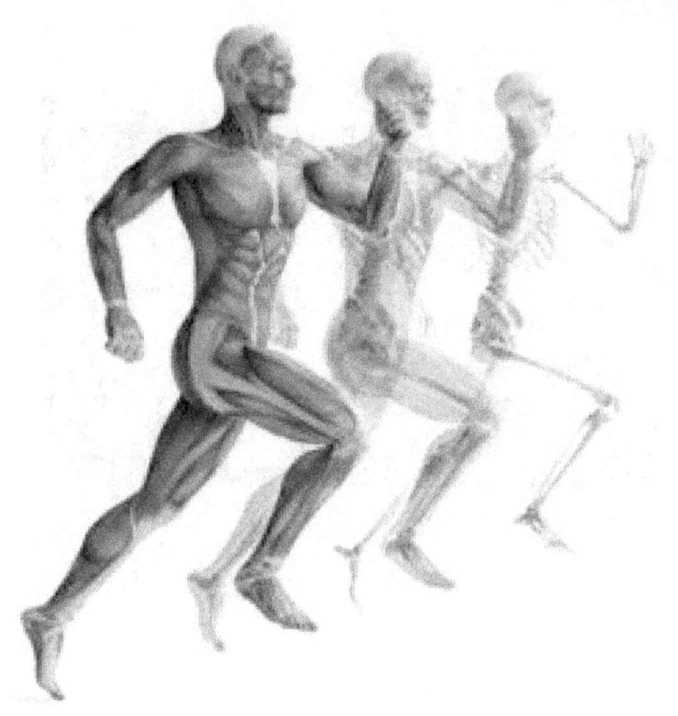

Handbook To Supreme Health & Fitness! ... At-Home Guide to Successfully Build Your God-Body!

*****

*****

Toned Muscles Work Better – Look Better

Weight training is one of the key elements of an overall fitness program. The training described here emphasizes a **general over-all physical fitness** rather than bodybuilding. **Everyone can become stronger. Everyone can see a marked difference after 6 to 10 weeks of conscientious strength training.**

Unused muscles ultimately atrophy, and even underused muscles quickly lose strength. The adage "use it or lose it" readily applies to muscles.

It is one thing to understand the importance of weight training. It is another thing to put that knowledge to work for you. **For muscles to become stronger, you need to demand more of them than their usual workload.**

When muscles are used often, they develop into **Good Muscle Tone. Good Muscle Tone means that even at rest, some muscle cells are always contracted.** Our skeletomuscular system can be enhanced when injury or problems from birth result in deviations to the sys- tem that produce stronger muscles and bones. Also, the muscular system is the organ system that can be altered most greatly by lifestyle choices.

Muscle tone: Constant partial contraction of muscle when the body is "in shape."

In a **Toned Muscle**, individual **Cells** sporadically **contract** and **relax**, causing no movement but **keeping the muscle taut. We can see muscle definition through the skin, due to this partial contraction**. Increased tone is an important benefit of regular exercise and not just for the 'buffed' look. **Toned muscles** are also **more effective** at **burning Energy**, which means that they use more ATP per gram than less-toned Muscle tissue.

People that are in-shape. can eat more without gaining weight because that continual, low-level contraction burns ATP. The summation is that a well-exercised body burns more calories in a day than an inactive body.

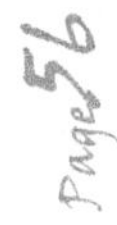

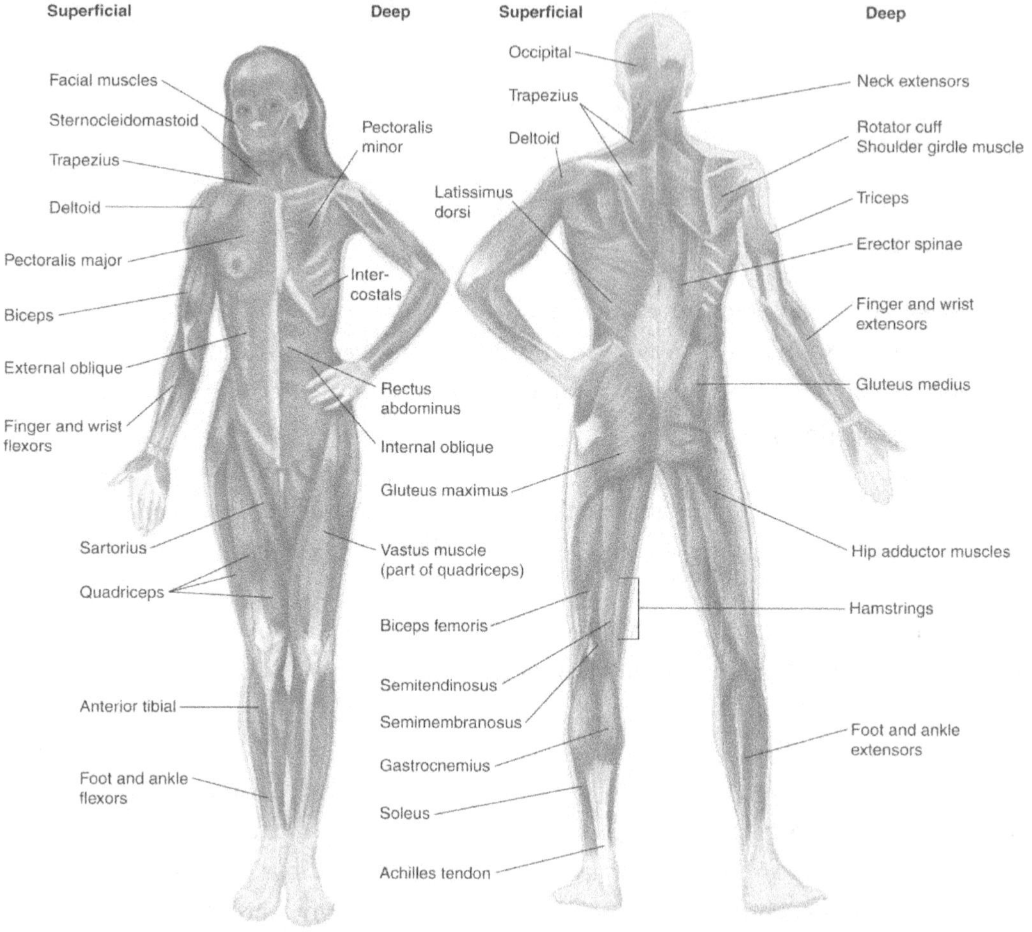

More Muscle May Reduce the Odds of Developing Diabetes

Researchers from the **University of California, Los Angeles** (UCLA), found that for each **10% increase in the skeletal muscle index** (the ratio of muscle mass to total body weight), **there was a corresponding 11% decline in insulin resistance and a 12% reduction in prediabetes** (a condition characterized by higher-than-normal blood sugar levels).

The findings represent a departure from the usual focus on just losing weight to improve metabolic health. Instead, this research suggests a role for maintaining fitness and building muscle. This is good news for many overweight people who experience difficulty in achieving weight loss, as any effort to get moving and keep fit should be seen as being beneficial. *Source*: Data from Srikanthan P., Karlamangla A. S. Relative muscle mass is inversely associated with insulin resistance and prediabetes. Findings from the third National Health and Nutrition Examination Survey. *Journal of Clinical Endocrinology and Metabolism* 2001; 96(9):2898-2903.

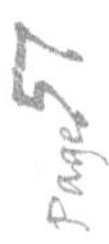

Scientists think the total number of muscle fibers is essentially set at birth, so how do we alter the appearance of this system?

We can do it through **muscle enlargement** or **hypertroph**y (*hyper* = <u>*above*</u>; *trophy* = <u>*to grow*</u>). Scientists believe **Hypertrophy** is caused by the **addition of new myofibrils** within the **endomysium** of individual muscle cells, which thickens individual **Myofibers**. Thus, **hypertrophic muscles** should have **thicker muscle cells**, packed with more **Sarcomeres** than non-**hypertrophic muscle cells**.

Exercise that requires muscle to contract to at least 75% of maximum tension will cause Hypertrophy. Bodybuilders use this knowledge to create their sculpted figures. Interestingly, aerobic exercises like cycling and dancing will not cause hypertrophy, but they still provide the cardiovascular and metabolic effects of increased muscle tone. Some people believe muscles can be built without any exercise at all.

Muscular Endurance

Muscular endurance describes **how long** or **how many times** (number of **repetitions**) you can **lift** and **lower** a given weight (often referred to as **resistance**). It can be assessed by determining the time or the number of repetitions of a particular exercise that can be performed.

For most people, developing muscular endurance is more important than muscular strength. Muscular endurance is usually more important in carrying out everyday activities.

Muscular Strength

As you lift and lower a weight, your muscle must generate enough force to move that weight. **Muscular strength** can be assessed by determining the amount of weight that can be lifted in one repetition of an exercise. **Strength can be developed by increasing the amount of weight that can be lifted in an exercise.**

Muscular Endurance: The ability of muscles to apply force repeatedly.

Muscular Strength: The force muscles can exert against resistance.

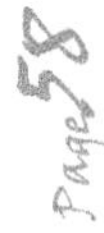

■   **To get stronger, use a few repetitions** (6–8) with maximum weight. The number of repetitions performed without stopping to rest is called a **set**.

■   **To gain endurance, use many repetitions** (12–15) with minimum weight to complete the set of repetitions.

Repetition (rep): A single lifting and lowering of the weight.

Set: Number of reps performed without stopping to rest.

Developing Different Types of Muscle Fiber

Muscles consist of many Muscle Fibers. Larger muscle fibers mean a **larger** and **stronger muscle (<u>hypertrophy</u>). When muscle fiber size diminishes**, the muscle fiber is said to **<u>atrophy</u>**.

Hypertrophy: Increase in bulk or size by thickening of muscle fibers.

Atrophy: Progressive loss (wasting) of muscle mass.

Two types of Muscle Fibers – Contraction Speed and Energy Source:

■   **Type I Slow-Twitch Fibers** do not contract as rapidly or strongly as fast-twitch fibers. They are **fatigue-resistant** and rely on **aerobic energy metabolism**.

■   **Type II Fast-Twitch Fibers** contract quickly and forcefully but **fatigue more rapidly** than slow-twitch fibers. They rely on **anaerobic energy metabolism**.

Endurance activities (i.e., jogging) use **slow-twitch fibers; power** and **strength activities** (i.e., sprinting) use **fast-twitch fibers.** *Weight training can increase the size and strength of both fiber types.*

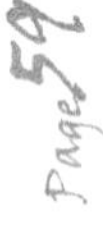

Everyone has both types of muscle fiber. Your genetics determine the proportion of each type of fiber in your body.

How Does Weight Training Change Body Composition and Metabolism?

Exercising the Muscles changes the Ratio of Fat to Muscle Fiber and speeds up weight loss. The **more muscle,** the **higher the metabolic rate** and the **more calories your body will burn on its own.**

It will be easier to keep your weight where you want it by eating right and exercising.

Exercising also slows degeneration of muscle and nerves with age. It keeps the bones strong, helping you to avoid osteoporosis. Being stronger when you are older keeps you from falling down as easily. Falls are the number one cause of injury for seniors.

Weight training keeps more of your motor nerves connected to the muscles they control. And you are better able to make quick and powerful moves.

Benefits of Muscular Strength and Endurance

Muscular strength and endurance are important components of physical fitness. **The benefits of strength and endurance training:**

■ **Improve** the capabilities of performing physical work, sports, recreation, and activities of daily living (e.g., walking).

■ **Raise** confidence by the way you look and help fight mild to moderate depression.

■ Help **prevent** osteoporosis (porous and less-dense bones), which makes the bones fragile and more vulnerable to fractures. **Strength training can slow bone loss and even help build bone.**

■ **Prevent** falls and fractures by improving balance and preserving power to correct missteps. By age 65, one in three people suffers a fall. Because bones also weaken over time, one out of every 20 of these falls causes a fracture, usually of the hip, wrist, or leg (National Safety Council 2007).

■ **Relieve** some of the load carried by the heart. **Strong muscles pluck oxygen and nutrients from the blood much more efficiently than weak ones do.** That means any activity requires less cardiac effort and puts less strain on your heart.

■ Help **control** blood glucose—**strong muscles are better at absorbing sugar in the blood and helping the body stay sensitive to insulin, which helps cells remove sugar from the blood.** In this way, strong muscles can help keep blood glucose levels in check, which in turn helps prevent or control type 2 diabetes.

■ **Increase** metabolism even while resting, resulting in more calories burned and, thus, helping keep weight within a healthy range.

■ Better manage stress and anxiety.

■ Improve posture.

■ Relieve arthritic pain and expand a limited range of motion.

■ Ease back and neck pain.

Gender Differences for Weight Training

Men are, on average, larger and stronger than women, because they have more muscle mass. But women have about the same strength in the lower body and only a small percentage less in the upper body. Why? Men have more androgens (hormones that cause facial hair, deep voice, and other sex-linked characteristics). Also, male muscles tend to activate faster, adding to muscle power.

Assessing Your Muscular Strength and Endurance

Muscular fitness is determined by assessing muscular strength and endurance.

■ **Muscular strength: Because muscular strength is specific to a muscle group, testing one group of muscles does not provide accurate information about the strength of other muscle groups.** For a comprehensive assessment, strength testing must involve several major muscle groups. Standard tests use free weights. The heaviest weight you can lift only one time through the full range of motion for a specific muscle group is considered your maximum strength for that muscle group.

■ **Muscular endurance: Muscular endurance is also specific to each muscle group**. Few tests of muscular endurance have been developed. Here at Supreme Health and Fitness we developed a bench-press test for muscular endurance using a standard weight. (Using the bench press to test strength is preferred by some experts. It is not a fair test for smaller, lighter individuals, however.)

F = Frequency

Completing a strength training routine two to three times per week can result in gains of muscle function and size. *The fastest gains are made in the first 4 to 8 weeks*; after that, gains are slower. Once you reach your goal, you can keep working out two to three times a week if you would like to make further gains. Or you can reduce your training to twice or even once a week to maintain the gains you have made.

Training can be done with "whole body" training sessions, exercising all muscle groups in the same session during the two to three times a week, or by using a "split-body" (upper body/lower body) routine, where a few muscle groups are trained during one session and the remaining muscle groups in the next. Both methods are effective as long as each muscle group is trained 2 to 3 days per week. ***Whichever routine is used, always allow at least 48 hours for muscles to recover between training workouts.***

I = Intensity

Intensity is the most critical part of resistance training. The basis of such training is **Progressive Overloading**. Progressive overloading strengthens individual muscle fibers and engages a larger proportion of available fibers in an activity. **This makes you stronger.**

Progressive Overloading: Increasing, from one session to another, the amount of weight you lift during a set.

Once you understand exactly how to do each exercise, choose a weight that allows you to do 12 repetitions. The last one or two repetitions should be difficult. If you cannot lift the weight at least eight times, use a lighter weight.

After a while, your muscles will gradually adapt to the weight you are using so you can do more repetitions. When you can comfortably perform 12 repetitions without completely tiring the muscle, it is time to increase the amount of weight.

Strength training focuses on tiring the muscles being worked. Once you have attained the desired level of strength and/or size, you can maintain that level of training—it is not necessary to increase the resistance, sets, or training sessions per week. **Strength may be maintained by training just 1 day per week if the resistance and intensity keeps constant.**

Resting for 2 to 3 minutes between sets produces the best strength gains in a general fitness program.

T = Time

Warm-up: Begin with a 5- to 10-minute warm-up. This will:

- **Prepare** the heart muscle and circulatory system for exercise

- **Warm** the muscles, making them more flexible

To warm-up, use low-intensity exercises (i.e., biking, stair-climbing, treadmill/jogging, or even low resistance with a high number of repetitions). When you begin to sweat, you are warmed up.

During the Workout: Strength training should:

- Enhance muscular fitness gradually over time to realize gains. You can do this several ways: (1) **increase** the number of repetitions, (2) increase **the** number of sets for a muscle group, or (3) **increase** the resistance by adding weight. Use only one of these options at a time to avoid injury.

- Have rhythmic movement, which means moving the weights smoothly without jerking.

- Involve moving the weights at a moderate to slow speed.

- Involve a full range of motion.

- Involve all of the major muscle groups (i.e., arms, shoulders, chest, back, legs).

- Not cause labored breathing (see the next section, T = Types of Resistance).

■ Change the exercises you perform for each muscle group every 4 to 8 weeks, even if you keep the same set and repetition routine. Changing exercises will **overload the muscles differently, increase** your **strength gains,** and alleviate boredom.

Exercise Order: The sequence of exercises during a workout can vary:

■ **Do large muscle group exercises before doing small muscle group exercises.**

■ Do **Multiple-Joint Exercises** (e.g., squats) before doing single-joint exercises (e.g., arms curl). *Why*? Because single-joint exercises fatigue the smaller muscle groups needed to perform multiple-joint exercises. An example of a **multiple-joint exercise** is the bench press, because your upper and lower arms move at the shoulder and elbow joints. An example of a **single-joint exercise** is a biceps curl, because only your lower arm moves at the elbow. To determine which exercises are multiple-joint exercises, watch and feel how many joints move while you perform the exercise.

■ **Lower-back** and **abdominal exercises should be done at the end of your workout because these muscles are used during other exercises for balance and posture.** If they are fatigued before doing the other exercises, you may not be able to do those exercises properly.

Multiple-Joint Exercise: An exercise in which two or more joints move together.

Cool-Down: Cool down for 2 to 5 minutes with a mild activity (e.g., walking, jogging, or cycling). Stretch after exercising—warm muscles stretch farther and are less likely to tear.

T = Types of Resistance Exercises

Resistance training can involve different types of equipment, such as free weights, machines with stacked weights or pneumatic resistance, and rubber bands. Each major muscle group (e.g., chest, shoulders, abdomen, back, legs, and arms) should be involved.

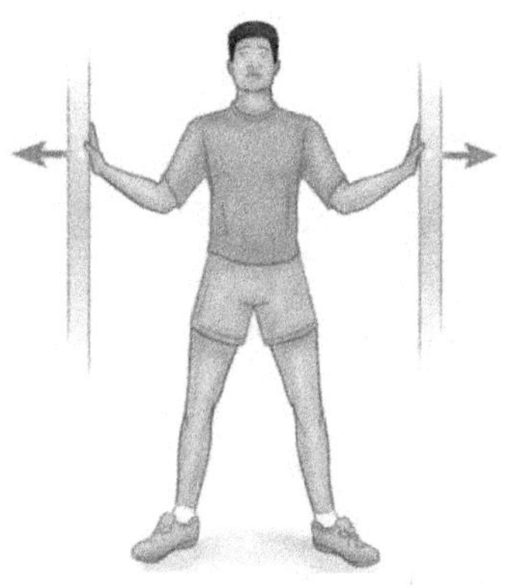

Isometric (Static) Exercises: **Isometric** (static) **exercise contracts muscle without changing muscle length** (does not involve joint or muscle movement).

■ Do these exercises against an immovable object (e.g., stand between door frames and push) to provide resistance.

■ **You can use isometric exercises to strengthen muscles after an injury or surgery**.

Advantages:

■ Require little or no equipment or expense

■ Low risk of muscle soreness

■ Can be done in a small space

■ Rapid strength improvement

Disadvantages:

■ Difficult to devise a full-body workout

■ Not very motivating

Isotonic Exercises

Isotonic (dynamic) **exercise contracts muscle in a way that changes muscle length** (involves muscle and joint movement). **Isotonic** is the most popular type of exercise for increasing muscle strength. It can be performed with weight machines. There are two kinds of muscle contractions:

■ **Concentric contractions** occur when the **muscle applies force** as it **shortens** and the joints move.

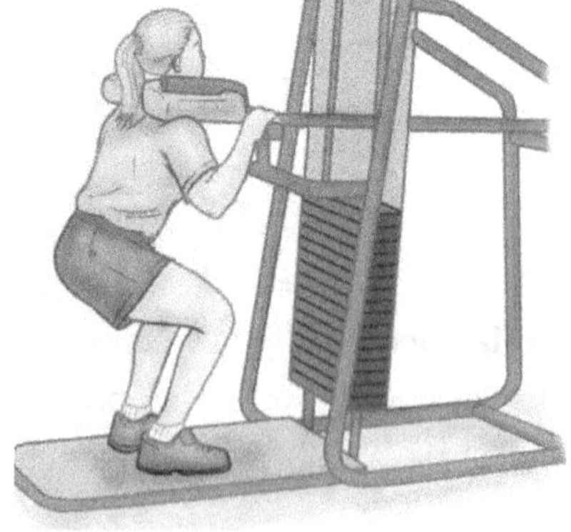

■ **Eccentric contractions** occur when the **muscle applies force** as it **lengthens** and the joints move.

For example, during an arm curl, the biceps muscle works concentrically as the weight is raised toward the shoulder and eccentrically as the weight is lowered.

Advantages:

■ Improve strength across the entire range of motion

■ Help improve joint flexibility

■ More motivating

Disadvantages:

■ Require more exercise equipment

■ Higher risk of muscle soreness

Isokinetic Exercises

Isokinetic exercise combines the advantages of both isometric and isotonic exercises. It uses special apparatus to provide a maximum resistance to the muscles, as in isometric exercise, but throughout the full range of motion, as in isotonic exercise. This equipment is often used by individuals who are in rehabilitation

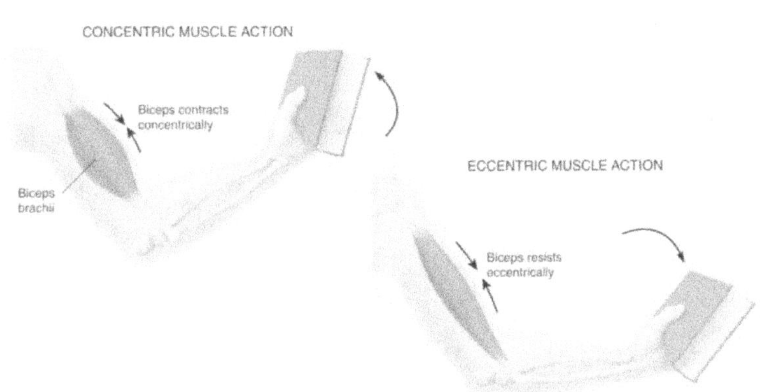

Two kinds of muscle contractions. Your muscles shorten during **Concentric action** (A) and lengthen during **Eccentric action** (B).

Isokinetic: Muscle contraction where the **maximum tension** is generated in the muscle as it contracts at a constant speed over the full range of motion of the joint.

Plyometric Exercises

Plyometrics involves doing abrupt, explosive movements, such as bounding on and off a box or jumping off a platform and immediately leaping upward. It develops quick-twitch muscle fibers but risks incurring injury. Do plyometric exercises only after you have developed well-conditioned muscles. These exercises may especially benefit some athletes.

Plyometrics: A form of training where muscles are subjected to rapid alternation of lengthening and shortening while resistance is continuously applied.

Example 1: Moderate-Intensity Activity and Muscle-Strengthening Activity

Sunday	Monday	Tuesday	Wednesday	Thursday	Friday	Saturday
30-minute brisk walk	30-minute brisk walk	30-minute brisk walk	Weight training	30-minute brisk walk	30-minute brisk walk	Weight training

Total: 150 minutes moderate-intensity aerobic activity

+ 2 days muscle-strengthening activity

Example 2: Vigorous-Intensity Activity & Muscle-Strengthening Activity

Sunday	Monday	Tuesday	Wednesday	Thursday	Friday	Saturday
	25-minute jog		25-minute jog and weight training		Weight training	25-minute jog

Total: 75 minutes vigorous-intensity aerobic activity

+ 2 days muscle-strengthening activity

Example 3: Moderate to Vigorous-Intensity Activity & Muscle Strengthening Activity

Sunday	Monday	Tuesday	Wednesday	Thursday	Friday	Saturday
30-minute brisk walk	15-minute jog	Weight training	30-minute brisk walk	Weight training	15-minute jog	30-minute brisk walk

Total: The equivalent of 150 minutes of moderate-intensity aerobic activity

+ 2 days muscle-strengthening activity

Moderate Aerobic Activity Routines

	Monday	Tuesday	Wednesday	Thursday	Friday	Saturday	Sunday	Physical Activity TOTAL
Example 1	30 minutes of brisk walking	30 minutes of brisk walking	Resistance band exercises	30 minutes of brisk walking	30 minutes of brisk walking	Resistance band exercises	30 minutes of brisk walking	150 minutes moderate-intensity aerobic activity AND 2 days muscle strengthening
Example 2	30 minutes of brisk walking	60 minutes of playing softball	30 minutes of brisk walking	30 minutes of mowing the lawn		Heavy gardening	Heavy gardening	150 minutes moderate-intensity aerobic activity AND 2 days muscle strengthening

Vigorous Aerobic Activity Routines

	Monday	Tuesday	Wednesday	Thursday	Friday	Saturday	Sunday	Physical Activity TOTAL
Example 3	25 minutes of jogging	Weight lifting	25 minutes of jogging	Weight lifting	25 minutes of jogging			75 minutes vigorous-intensity aerobic activity AND 2 days muscle strengthening
Example 4	25 minutes of swimming laps		25 minutes of running	Weight training	25 minutes of singles tennis	Weight training		75 minutes vigorous-intensity aerobic activity AND 2 days muscle strengthening

Mix of Moderate and Vigorous Aerobic Activity Routines

	Monday	Tuesday	Wednesday	Thursday	Friday	Saturday	Sunday	Physical Activity TOTAL
Example 5	30 minutes of water aerobics	30 minutes of jogging	30 minutes of walking Yoga		30 minutes of brisk walking	Yoga		90 minutes moderate-intensity aerobic activity AND 30 minutes vigorous-intensity aerobic activity AND 2 days muscle strengthening
Example 6	45 minutes of doubles tennis Weight lifting	Rock climbing			30 minutes of vigorous hiking		45 minutes of doubles tennis	90 minutes moderate-intensity aerobic activity AND 30 minutes vigorous-intensity aerobic activity AND 2 days muscle strengthening

Four health risk behaviors—lack of physical activity, poor nutrition, tobacco use, and excessive alcohol consumption—are responsible for much of the illness and death related to chronic diseases. Seven out of 10 deaths among Americans each year are from chronic diseases. Heart disease, cancer, and stroke account for more than 50% of all deaths each year.

A Centers for Disease Control study finds that people can live longer if they practice one or more healthy lifestyle behaviors—not smoking, eating a healthy diet, getting regular physical activity, and limiting alcohol consumption. Not smoking provides the most protection from dying early from all causes.

People who engaged in all four healthy behaviors were 63% less likely to die early from cancer, 65% less likely to die early from cardiovascular disease, and 57% less likely to die early from other causes compared to people who did not engage in any of the healthy behaviors. *Source*: Data from Ford E.S., et al., Low-risk lifestyle behaviors and all-cause mortality. *American Journal of Public Health* 2011. 101(10): 1922–1929.

Where Should You Exercise?

At a Health Club/Gym: Advantages:

- Availability of professional supervision and trainers

- Many exercise options, including aerobic options

At Home: Advantages:

- Convenient: no concerns about appearance, travel time, parking, gym hours

- Private: avoids strangers, not intimidating if you feel weak and awkward

- No waiting in line; no noise from loud music and talking

- Cleaner: the germs on the bench and bars are yours

- Less expensive: no monthly payments for health club membership

Weight Machines: Circuit Training:

Circuit training combines aerobic and strength exercises.

- Each exercise station takes 30 to 45 seconds to do.

- Stations alternate between upper and lower body exercises.

- The circuit is repeated two or more times per session.

- Do a circuit-training workout three times each week for aerobic conditioning and moderate increases in strength.

Proper Free-Weight Lifting Techniques:

- Keep weights as close to your body as possible.

- Do most of the lifting with your legs.

- Keep your hips and buttocks tucked in.

- Keep your hands dry.

- Wear gloves to prevent calluses and blisters.

- Wrap your thumbs around the bar when gripping it.

- When picking up a weight from the ground, keep your back straight and your head level or up.

- Warm up before lifting.

- Use **spotters** and **collars** with free weights.

- Start slowly and progress gradually.

- Perform exercises smoothly and with good form.

- Lift or push the weight forcefully during the active phase of the lift and then lower it slowly with control.

- Perform all lifts through the full range of motion to reduce the chance of injury and soreness. Do not lock (fully straighten) your knees or elbows when involved in an exercise, because this practice stresses the joint.

- Exhale when exerting the greatest force, and inhale when moving the weight into position for the active phase of the lift.

- Rest between sets if you perform more than one set of each exercise.

- If you feel pain during an exercise, stop immediately. Continue only if the pain subsides, but reduce the amount of weight.

- Soreness the next day is normal when first starting to exercise or when increasing the amount of weight you lift.

- Cool down after a workout.

Improper Free-Weight Lifting Techniques: Do not do the following:

- Bend at the waist with legs straight;

- Twist your body while lifting;

- Jerk weights; lift smoothly and slowly;

- Bounce weights against your body during an exercise;

- Arch your back when lifting a weight;

- Lift beyond the limits of your strength; or

- Hold your breath when lifting.

*****

American College of Sports Medicine: *http://www.acsm.org*

Exercise Prescription: *http://www.exrx.net*

National Strength and Conditioning Association: *http://www.nsca-cc.org*

National Council of Strength and Fitness: *http://www.ncsf.org*

Physician and Sports Medicine: *http://www.physsportsmed.com*

*References and Suggested Readings

———. Prescription of resistance training for health and disease. *Medicine and Science in Sports and Exercise* 1999; 31:38–45.

American College of Sports Medicine (ACSM). The recommended quantity and quality of exercise for developing and maintaining cardiorespiratory and muscular fitness and flexibility in healthy adults. *Medicine and Science in Sports and Exercise* 1998; 30:975–991.

American College of Sports Medicine. Quantity and Quality of Exercise for Developing and Maintaining Cardiorespiratory, Musculoskeletal, and Neuromotor Fitness in Apparently Healthy Adults: Guidance for Prescribing Exercise. *Medicine and Science in Sports and Exercise*. DOI: 10.1249/MSS.0b0138213fefb

Braill P. A., et al. Muscular strength and physical function. *Medicine and Science in Sports and Exercise* 2000; 32:412–416.

Ebben W. P. and Jensen R. L. Strength training for women. *Physician and Sports Medicine* 1998; 26:86.

Feigenbaum M. S. and Pollock M. L. Strength training: Rationale for current guidelines for adult fitness programs. *Physician and Sports Medicine* 1997; 25:44.

Garber, C. E., et al. Quantity and quality of exercise for developing and maintaining cardiorespiratory, musculoskeletal, and neuromotor fitness in apparently healthy adults: Guidance for prescribing exercise. *Medicine in Science and Sports and Exercise* 2011; 43(7):1334–1359.

National Safety Council. *Inquiry Facts*. Itasca, IL: National Safety Council, 2007.

Stamford B. Weight training basics. Part 1: Choosing the best options. *Physician and Sports Medicine* 1998; 26:115–116.

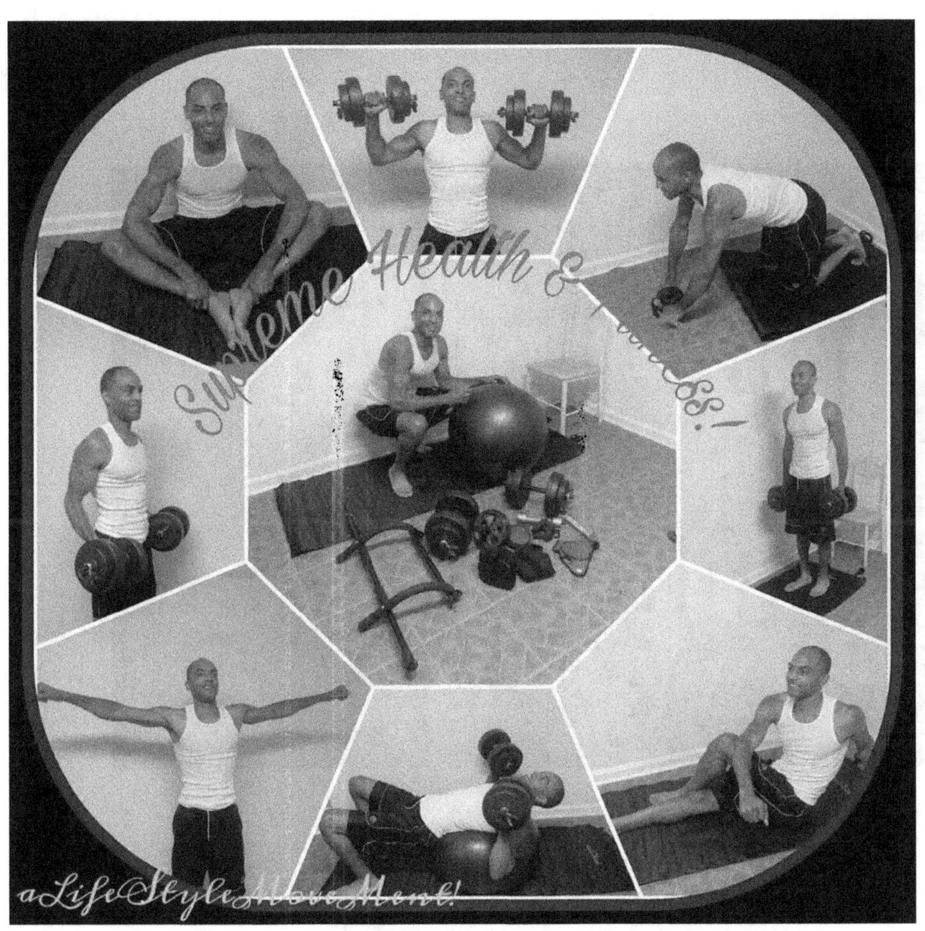
Supreme Health & Fitness!
a LifeStyle MoveMent!

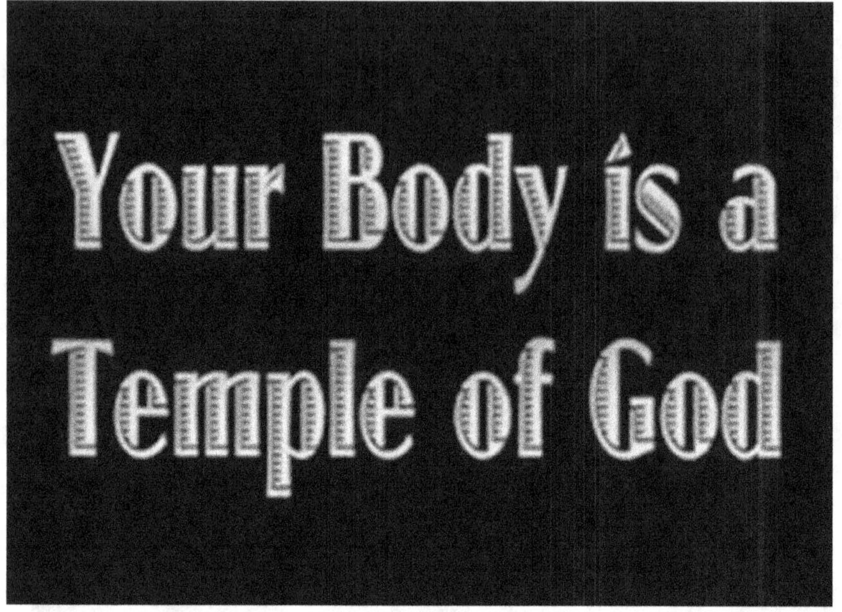

*****

Building Muscloskeletal Strength and Definition ... Creating Your God-Body

Total Body ... Using Your Own Body Weight!

Activity 1: Supreme Push-up

...Thiis is Activity isone of our Natural Easily performed and most Effective Upper Body Activities because it incorporates almost every Muscle-Tendon group in this region ... By adding the Ball – the Intensity level increases as well as the Results!

Push-ups

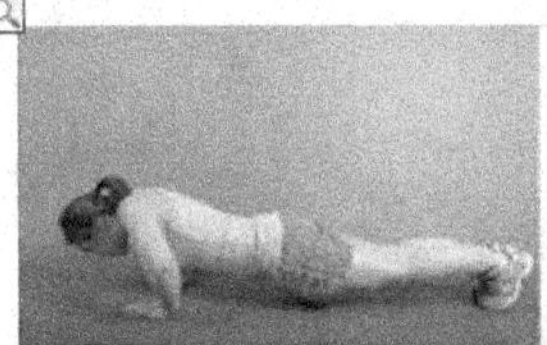 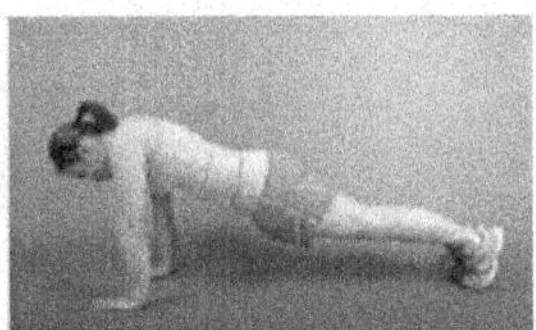

Modified Push-up

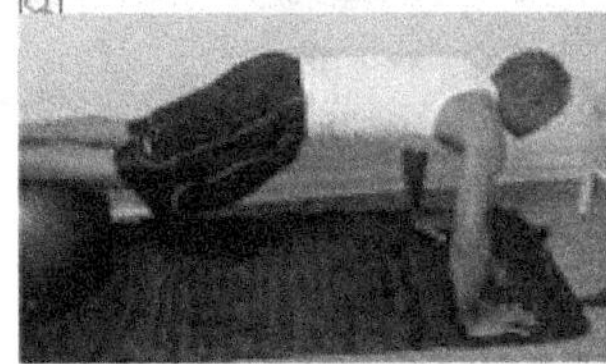 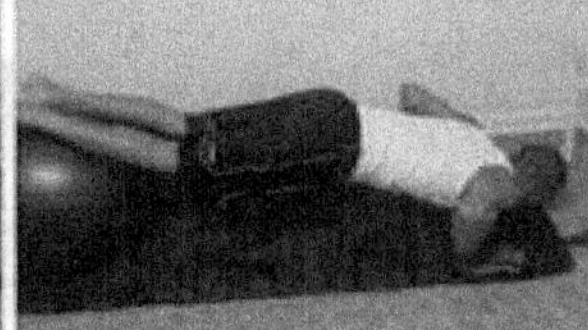

Muscles developed: triceps, deltoids, pectoralis major, abdominals, and erector spinae

- Keep your back as straight as possible. Flex your elbows. Lower your body until it almost touches the floor; pause momentarily, and then raise yourself back up to the starting position and repeat.

- You can use a bench, chair, or stairway to support your hands, rather than the floor. Increase resistance by having someone push down on your way up.

- If you are unable to do push-ups as described, do modified push-ups by placing your lower body on your knees rather than on your feet.

Activity 2: Supreme Body Dip!

Modified Dip

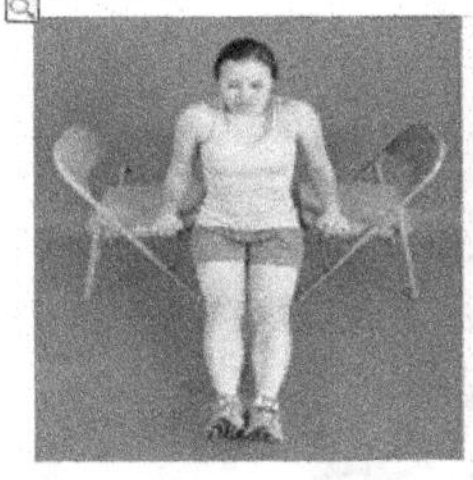 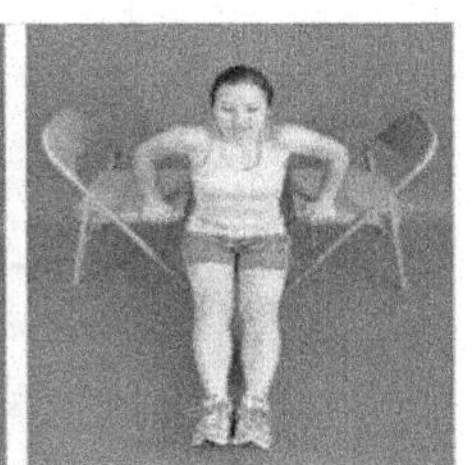

Muscles developed: triceps, deltoids, and pectoralis major

- Place your hands on opposite chairs or use parallel bars.

- With your knees slightly bent, dip down to at least a 90° angle at the elbow joint, pause momentarily, and then raise yourself back up to the starting position. Repeat. Increase resistance by having someone push down on your way up.

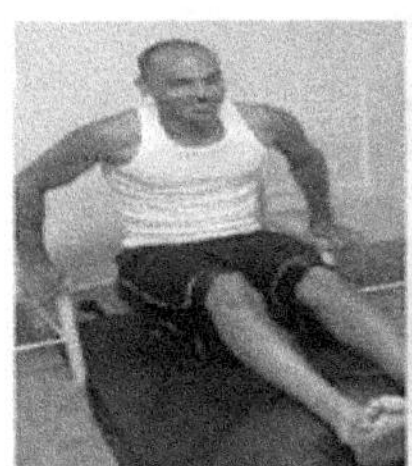 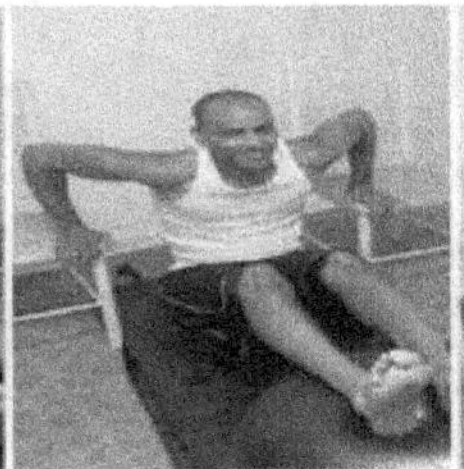 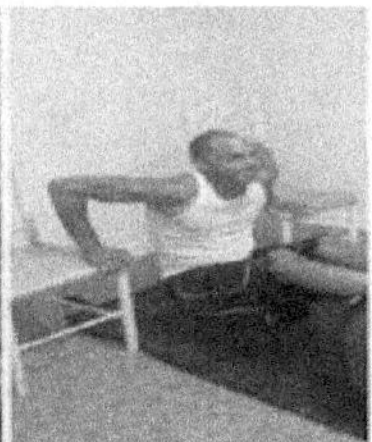

This is a great at-home Activity to help Tighten up the Triceps (Back-Arms) area ... with benefits to the Deltoids and Pecs!

Adding the Ball allows you to Increase both the Intensity and the RESULTS!

Activity 3: Building a Strong Back Supreme Body Pull-Ups!

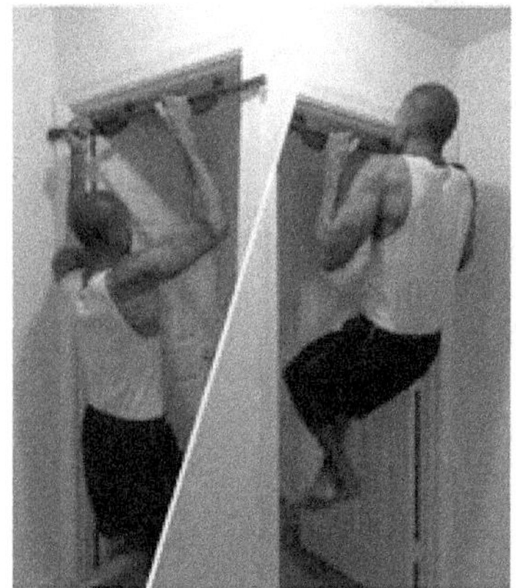
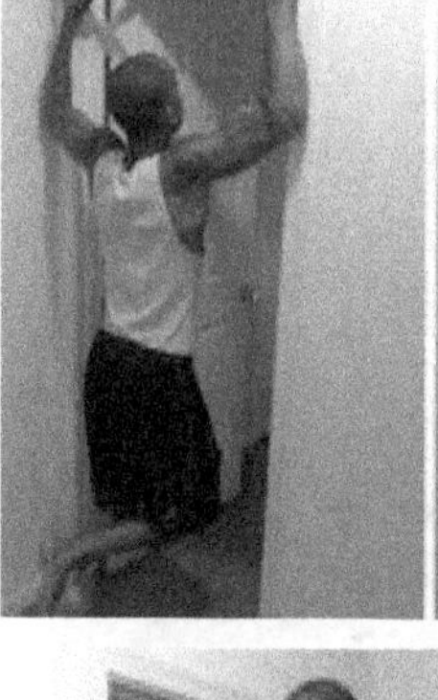
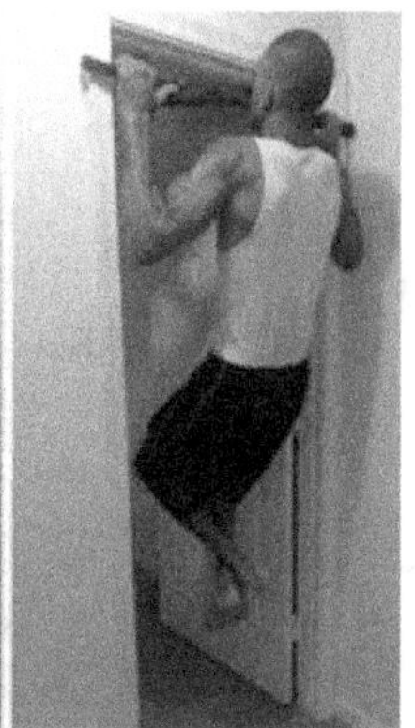

This is one of my Favorite Activities ... You really Feel an Increase in Strength and Development in almost Youe entire Upper Body! With the Pull-up bar, there are 4 main hand positions that are used to achieve the desired results — Under-Hand and Over-Hand, Wide and Hammer Grips!

The two main Muscle groups that are Actuvated re the Trapezius and Latissimus Dorsi which are the major Muscle groups of the Upper Back.

Each position works a different portion of these Miscle groups. The Deltiods, Rhomboids, Teres Major & Minor, Infraspinatus and Erector Spinae conclude the Muscles groups activated for creating a Supreme Back!

****

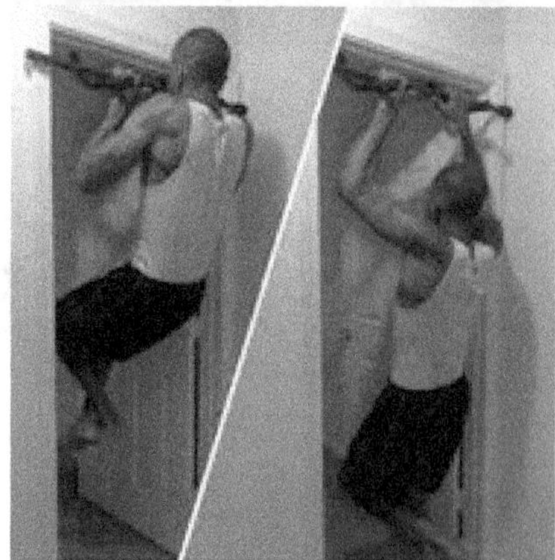

Activity 4: Supreme Wheel of Power

This is an excellent Activity to Build, Strengthen and Maintain a Strong Core and Solid Center of Gravity! Eventhough this is a Core Strengthening Activity, by the 5th rep, You will Feel a Total Body Activation ... even in Your TOES!!

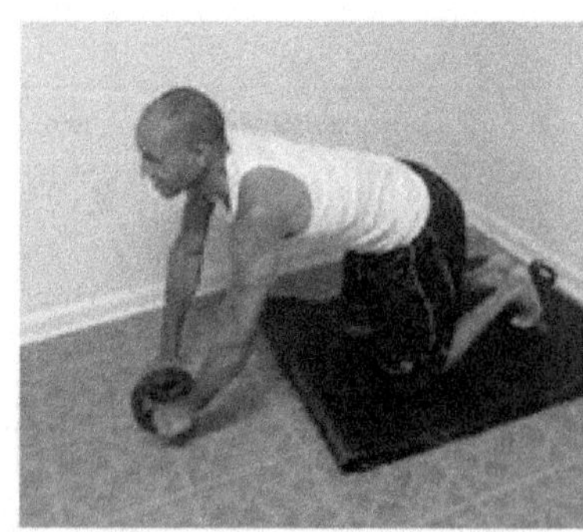
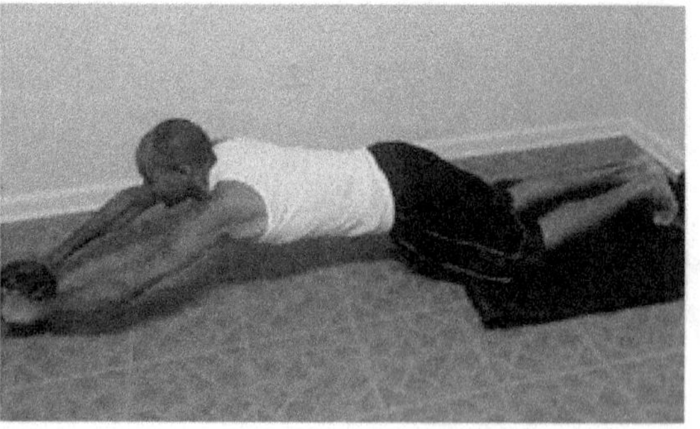

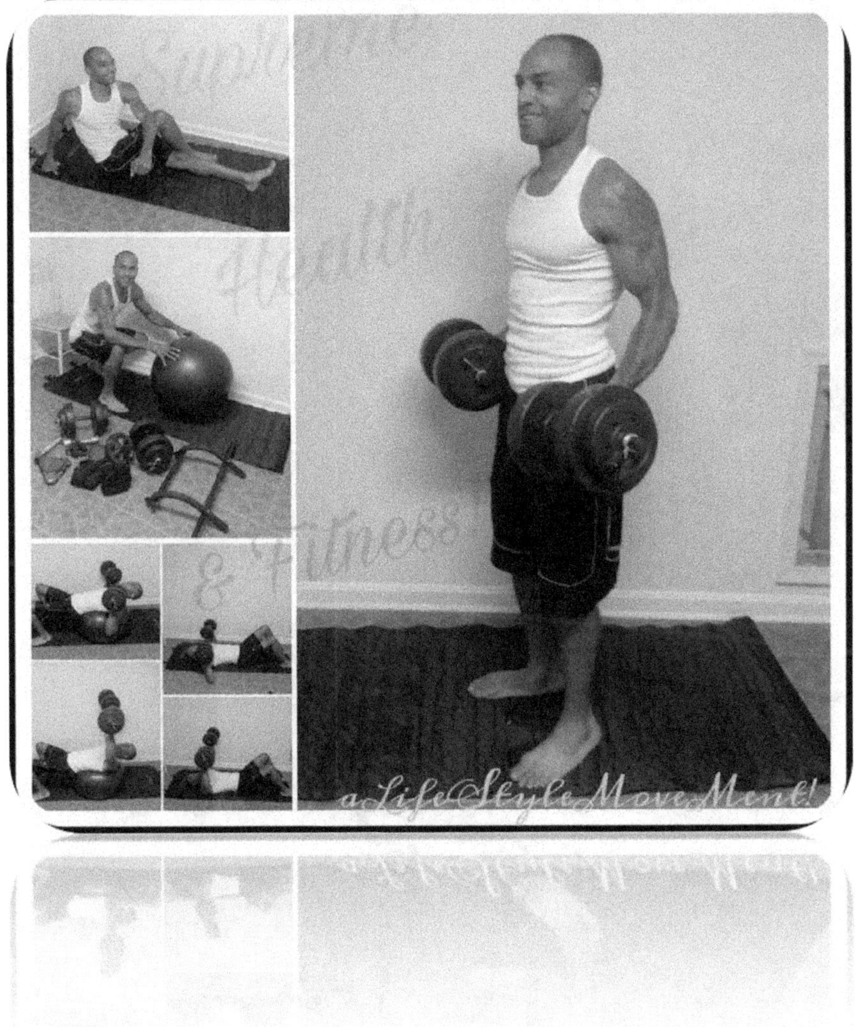
a LifeStyle MoveMent!

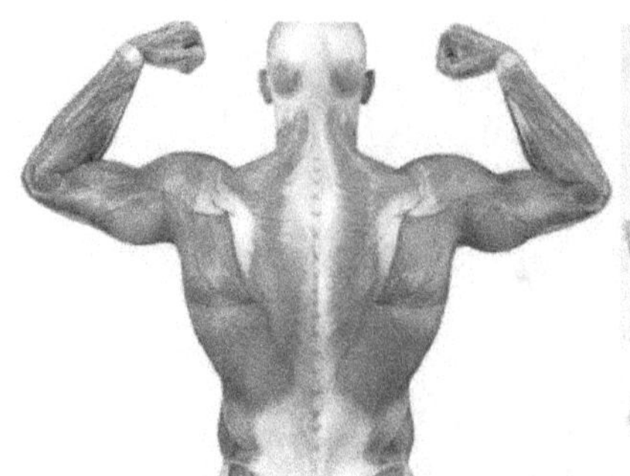

What God Says About My Body

*Total Body ...

Training with Weights

Activity 1: Supreme Bench Press or Barbell Press

Bench Press

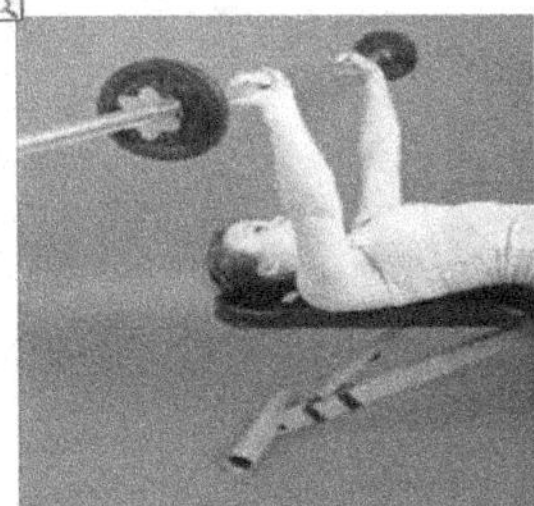 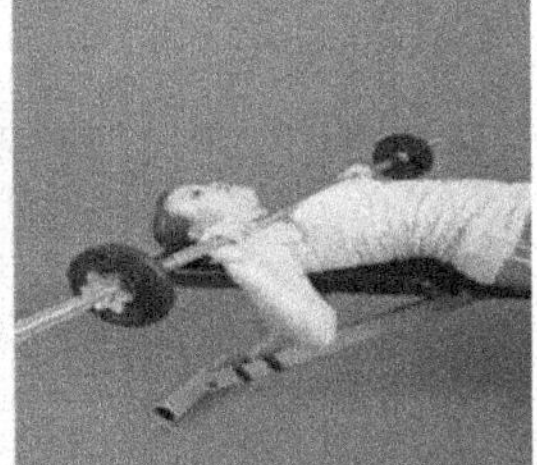

Muscles developed: pectoralis major, triceps, deltoids

- Lie facing up on a bench, your feet flat on the floor, with your head, shoulders, and buttocks pressed down firmly.
- Grip the bar with your hands about shoulder width apart or slightly wider. Push the bar from a low point on your chest to a high point over your chin.
- Extend your arms, pause momentarily, and then lower them slowly. Repeat.
- **Do not** arch your back or raise your buttocks during lifting.
- **Do not** bounce the bar off of your chest.

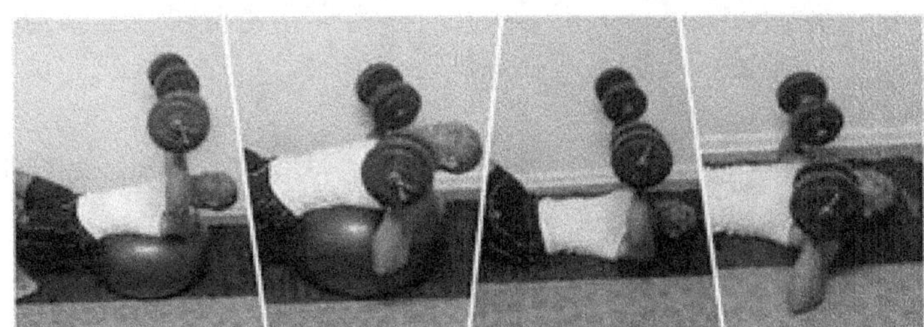

If you don't have access to a weight bench and/or barbell ... No Worries ... You can successfully perform this Activity with the same intensity with an Exercise Ball and dumb-bells or simply lie flat on the floor.

*****

Activity 2: Power Boulder Shoulders Supreme Military Press!

Shoulder (military press)

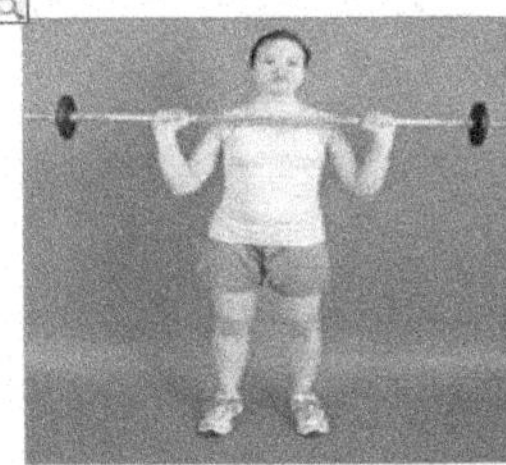 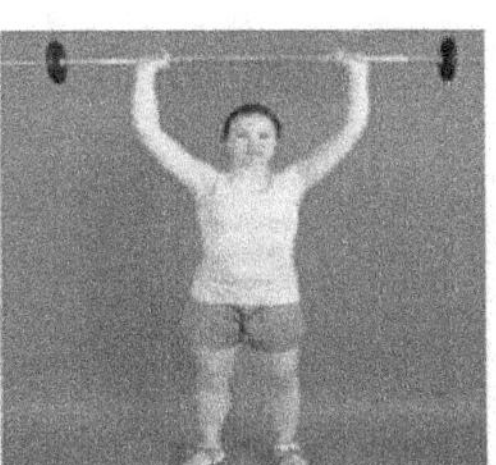

Muscles developed: deltoids, triceps, trapezius

Stand or sit with your feet shoulder-width apart. Keep your eyes straight ahead and your back straight. Place your hands shoulder-width apart. Push the bar overhead to arm's length, pause, and then slowly lower it. Repeat.

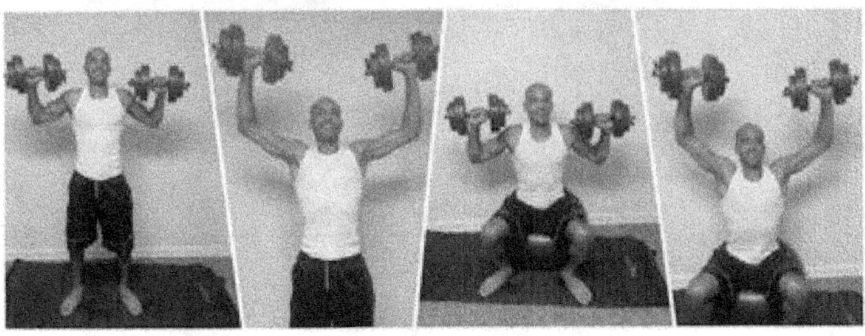

If you don't have a barbell, this Activity can be performed with dumb-bells for the same Intensity and Results!

For additional Intensity, you can perform this Activity on a Ball, Balancing and Activating and Strengthening Your CORE.

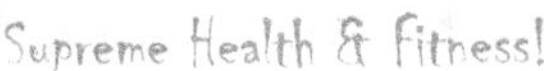

Activity 3: Building Your Strong Guns Supreme Biceps Curls!

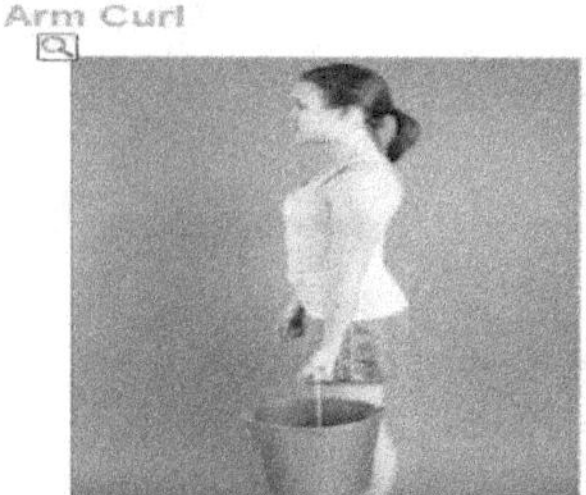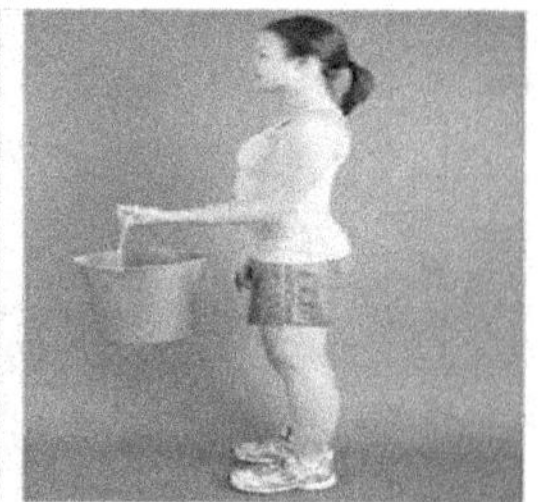

Arm Curl

Muscles developed: biceps

- Use a palms-up grip to raise a bucket filled with rocks, sand, or dirt.

- Start with one arm completely extended. Curl up your arm as far as possible, pause momentarily, and then extend your arm back to the starting position and repeat.

- Repeat the exercise with your other arm.

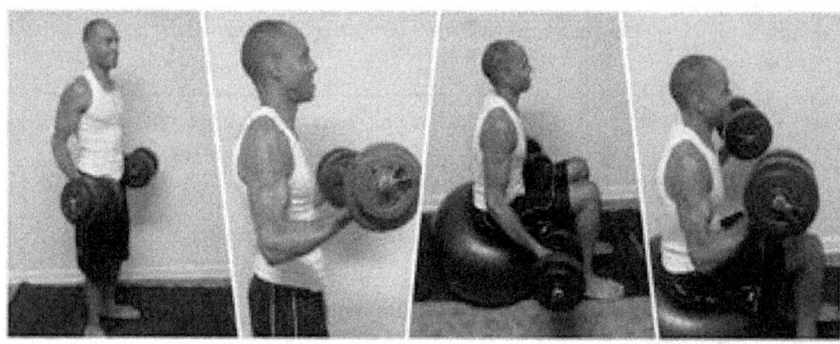

Because these are At-Home Activities, you can get the necessary Resistance needed to Strengthen and Activate Muscle Growth from any household items.

Using a Ball to create Balancing, Strengthening to your CORE and it adds a degree of Intensity for more Results!

*****

Activity 4: Arm Tightening Supreme Triceps Curls!

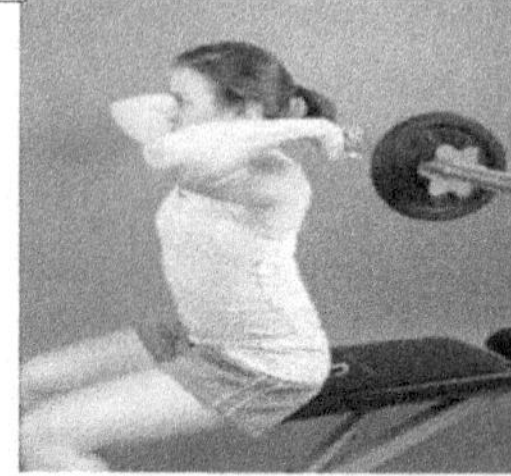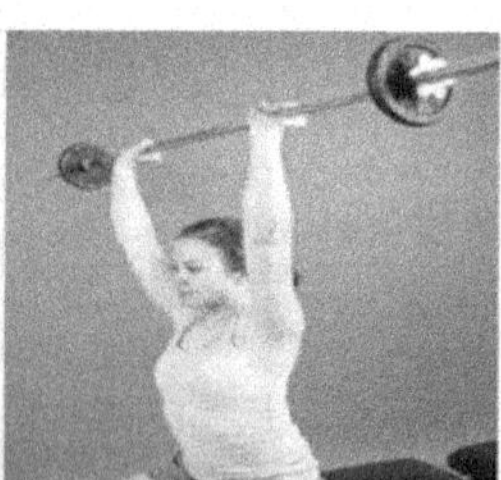

Triceps Curl

Muscles developed: triceps

Sit erect with your elbows and palms facing up, the bar resting behind your neck on your shoulders. Your hands should be shoulder-width apart. Slowly curl the weight overhead, pause, and slowly lower it. Repeat.

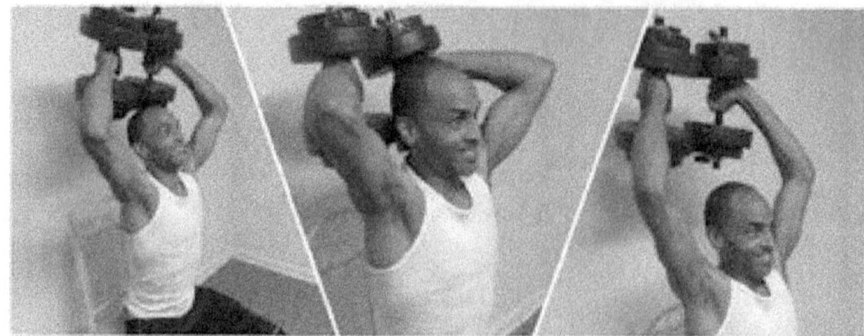

This Activity can be performed Successfully with a chair and dumb-bells.

Using dumb-bells add a level of Intensity and increase the Results!

Activity 5: Supreme Lateral Raise!

Lateral Raise

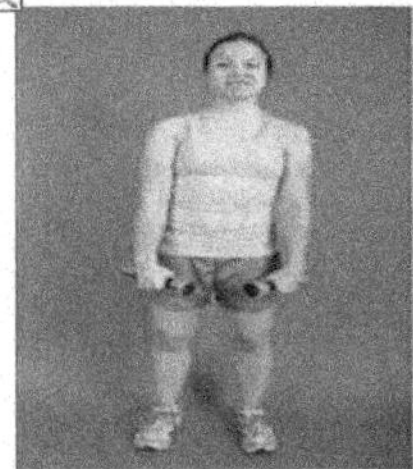 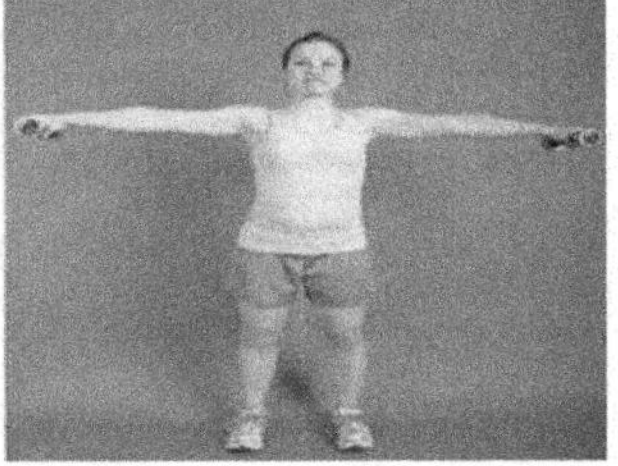

Muscles developed: deltoids

- Start with a dumbbell in each hand and feet apart.
- Slowly lift weights with elbows slightly bent.
- Lift weights until level with shoulders.
- Slowly lower the weights to starting position.

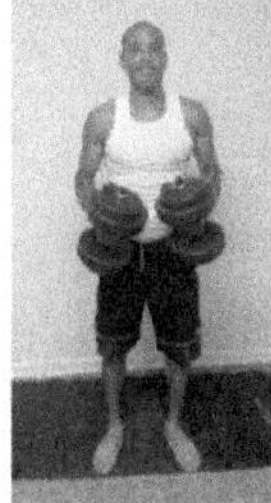 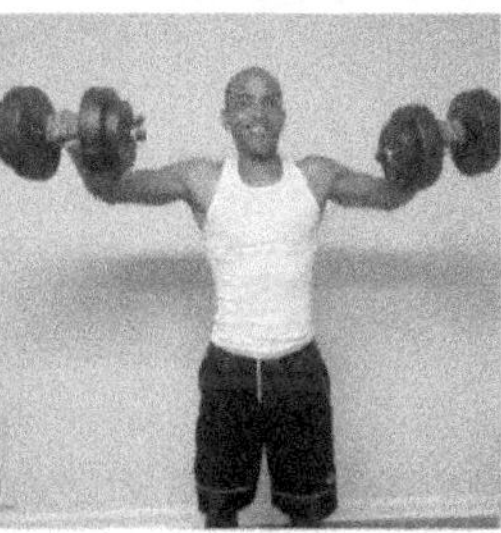 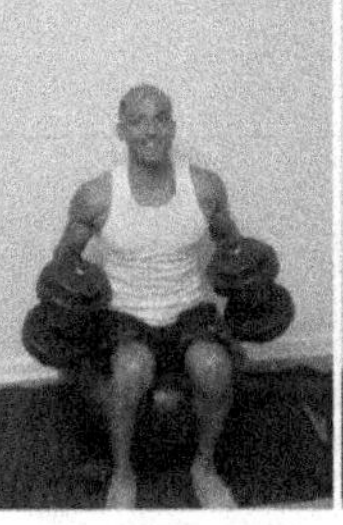 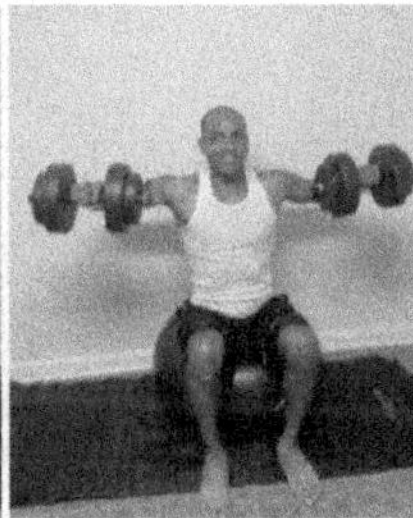

This Activity can be easily accomplished with dumb-bells.

You can add the exercise ball to increase resistance and add Core Strengthening!

Activity 6: Supreme Standing Rows!

Upright Rowing

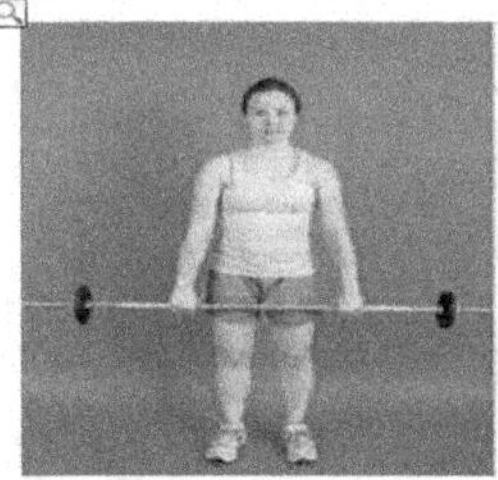 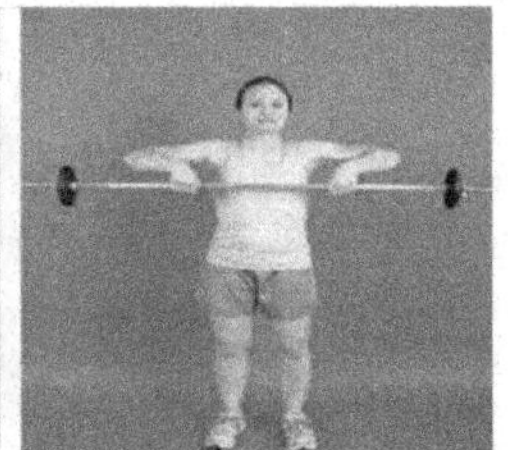

Muscles developed: trapezius, deltoids, biceps

- In a standing position, grip the bar with palms down and 4 to 8 inches apart.
- Keep your eyes straight ahead and chest high.
- Raise the bar until it reaches chin height, pause momentarily, and then lower slowly. Repeat.
- Keep your weight close to the front of your body, and make sure that your elbows stay higher than your hands.

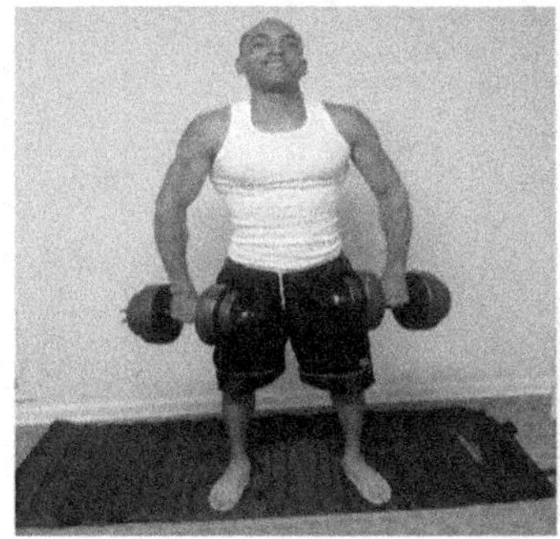 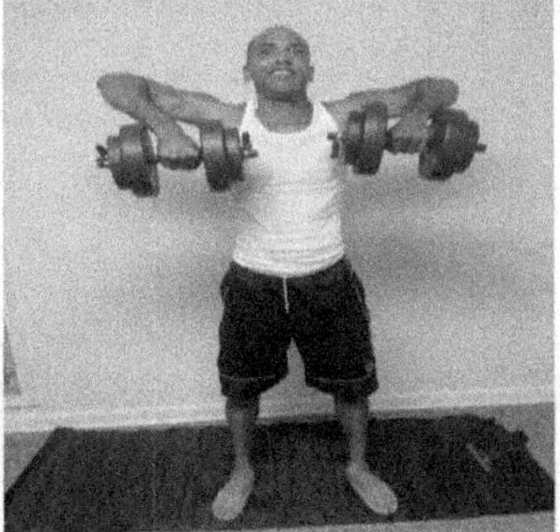

You can successfully perform this Activity with dumb-bells and get the same resistance with same results.

Dumb-bells can add a wider range-of-motion and be add a level of resistance by adding Balance training.

Activity 7: Supreme Half Squat!

Half Squat

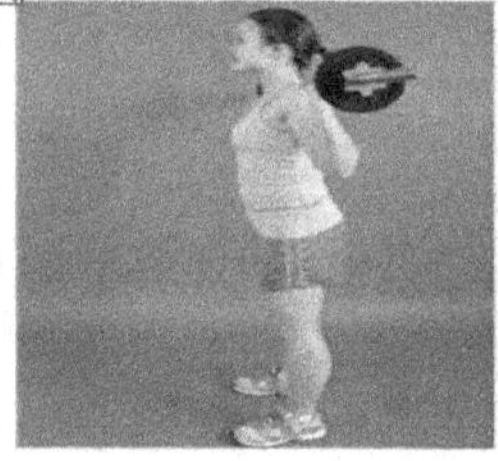 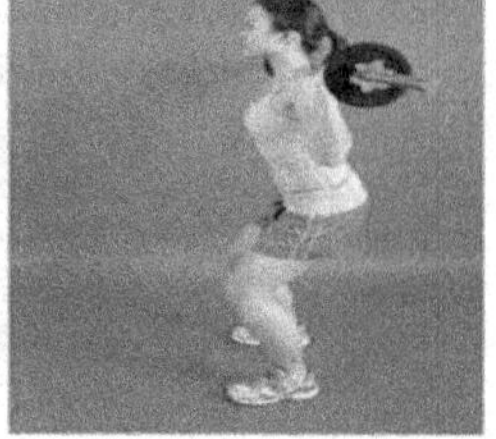

Muscles developed: quadriceps, gluteus maximus, hamstrings, gastrocnemius

- Stand erect with the bar resting on your trapezius muscles (shoulder muscles), not your neck.
- Use an overhand grip, with your hands and feet spread shoulder-width part.
- Lower your weight by bending at the knees to a 90° angle, pause, and slowly return to an upright position. Repeat.
- Keep your back straight; do not bend forward at the waist.
- **Do not** squat beyond halfway or bounce at the bottom.
- Place a bench behind you so that you can sit down if you lose your balance. Use spotters.

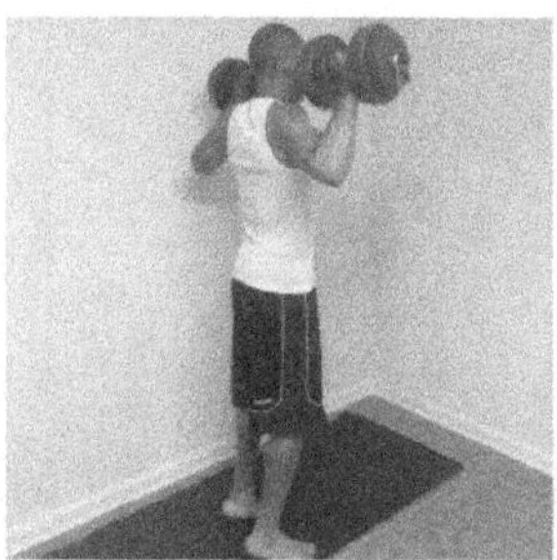 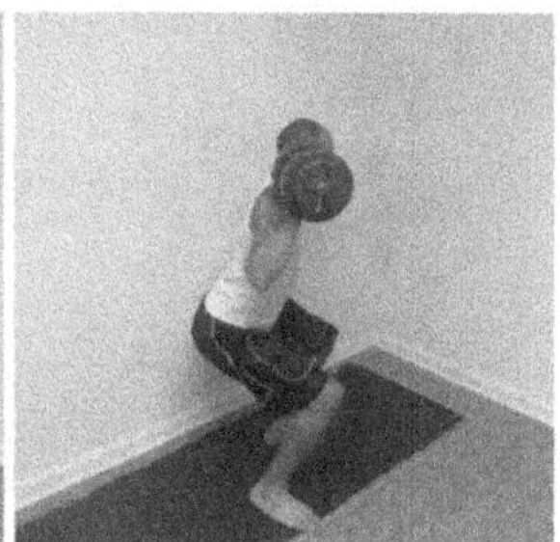

If you don't have access to a barbell set, you can add the same resistance with dumb-bells.

Dumb-bells can be easier to use, present less strain on your Rotator Cuff and allow for a better range-of-motion.

Activity 9: Supreme Lunge

Lunge

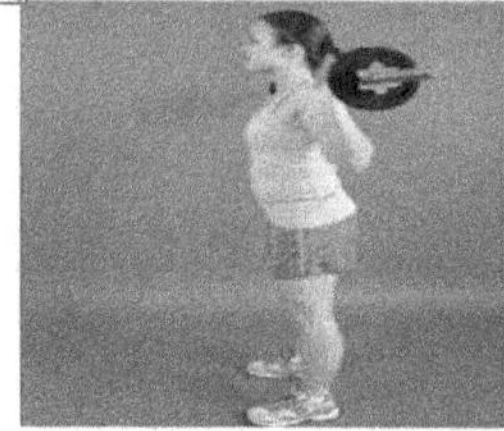 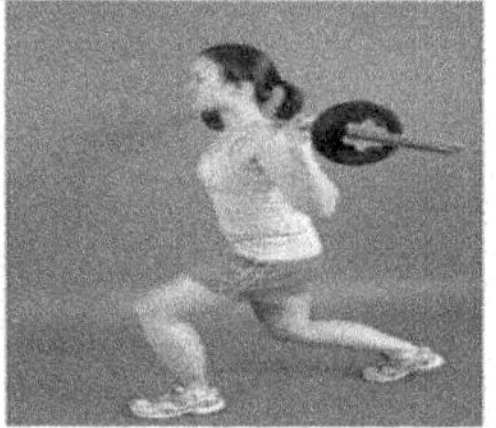

Muscles developed: thigh, gluteal

- Place the barbell behind your head or use a dumbbell in each hand.
- Keep the weight of the bar mainly on your trapezius muscles, not your neck.
- Your hands should be shoulder-width apart.
- Keep your head up and look forward, with your back straight.
- Slowly take a step forward and allow your leading leg to drop so that it is nearly parallel with the floor. The lower part of your leg should be nearly vertical and your back should be kept upright.
- Pause momentarily, and then take a stride with your other leg to return to a standing position.
- Repeat with your other leg.

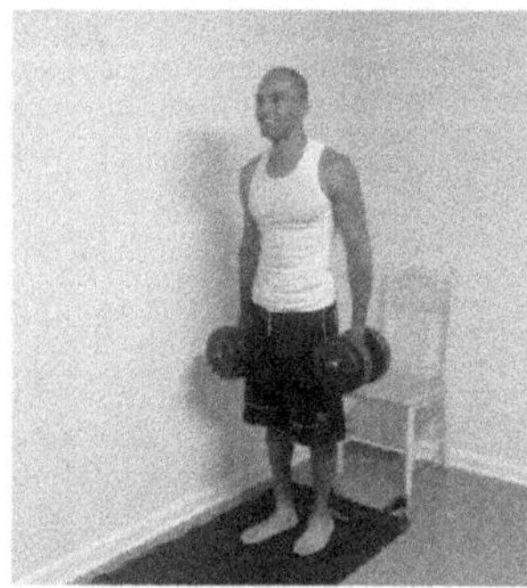 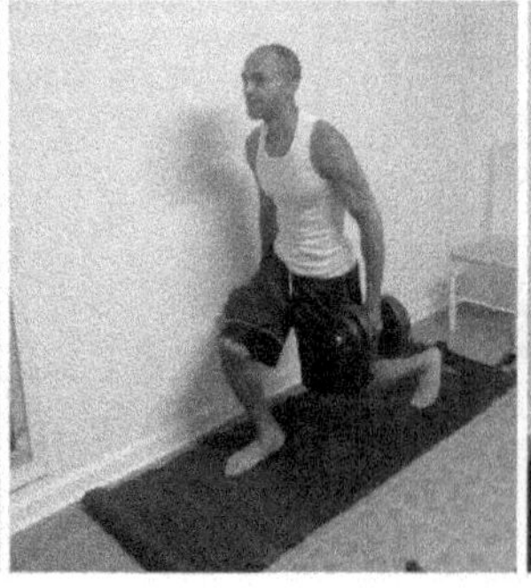 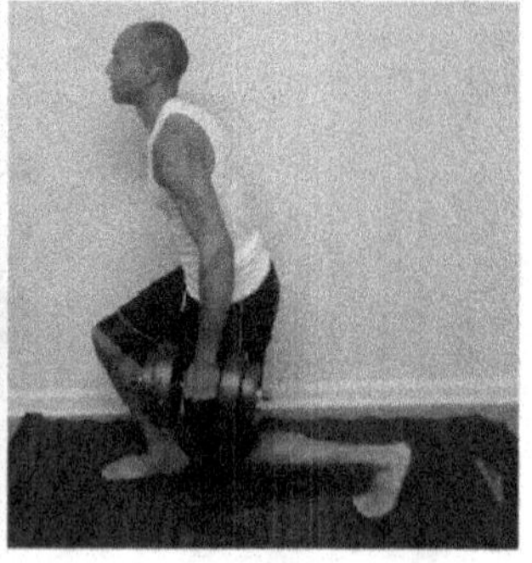

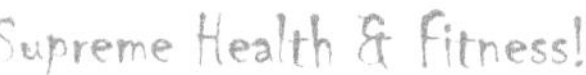

Activity .8: Supreme Heel/Calf Raise

Heel Raise

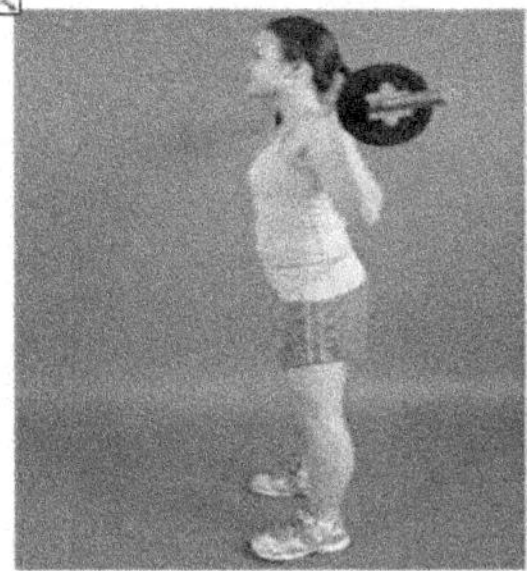 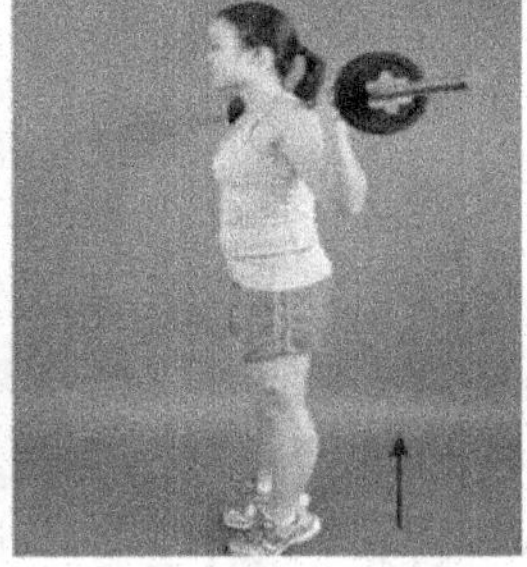

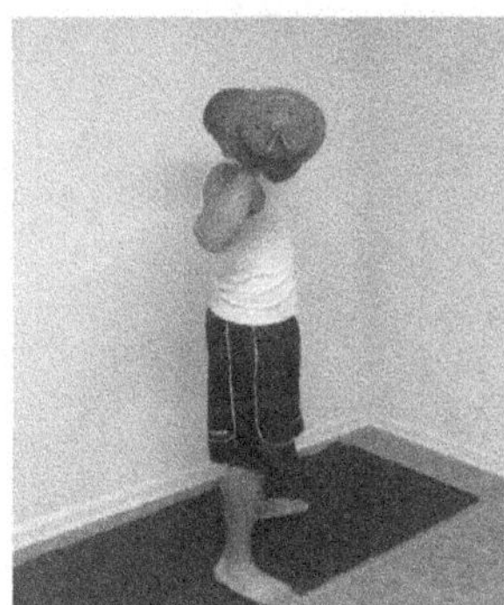 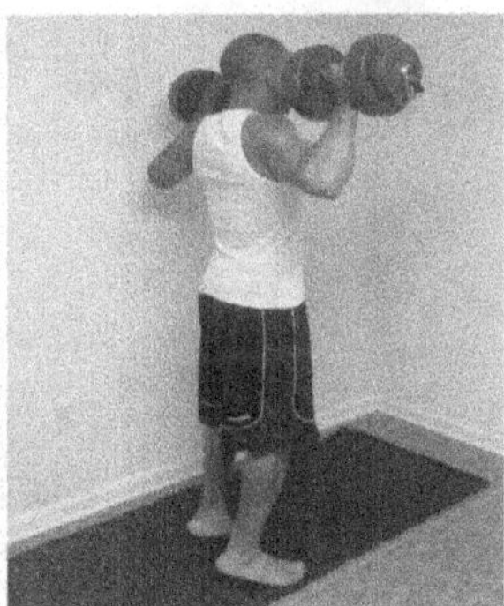

Muscles developed: gastrocnemius, soleus

- Stand erect with your hands and feet spread shoulder-width apart.

- Hold the bar resting on your shoulders (see half squat) or hold a dumbbell in each hand. Use an overhand grip.

- With your feet flat on the floor, slowly push down on your toes while lifting your heels as high as possible, pause momentarily, and then lower slowly. Repeat.

- You can also do this exercise by placing the front one-third of each foot on the edge of a bottom stair or wood block, with the backs of your feet hanging off.

This Activity can be Successfully completed with dumb-bells.

Using dumb-bells adds an increased level of by adding Stability Training which can help Strengthen and Improve your Core!

Supreme Health & Fitness!

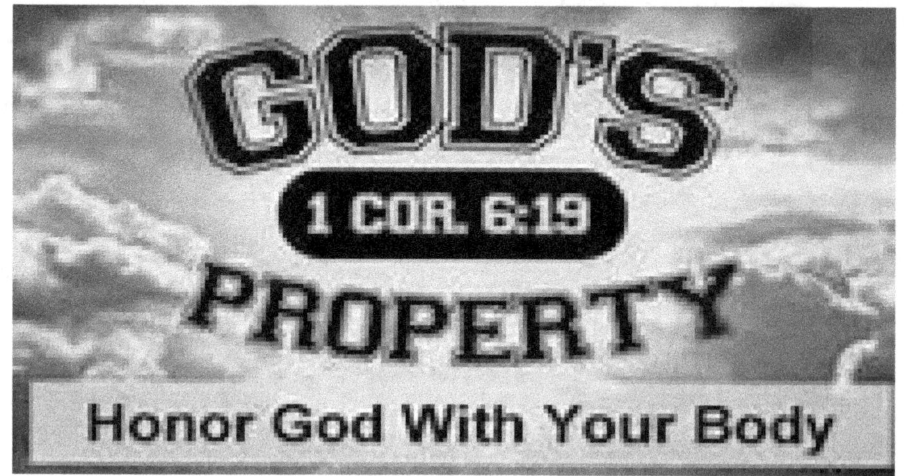

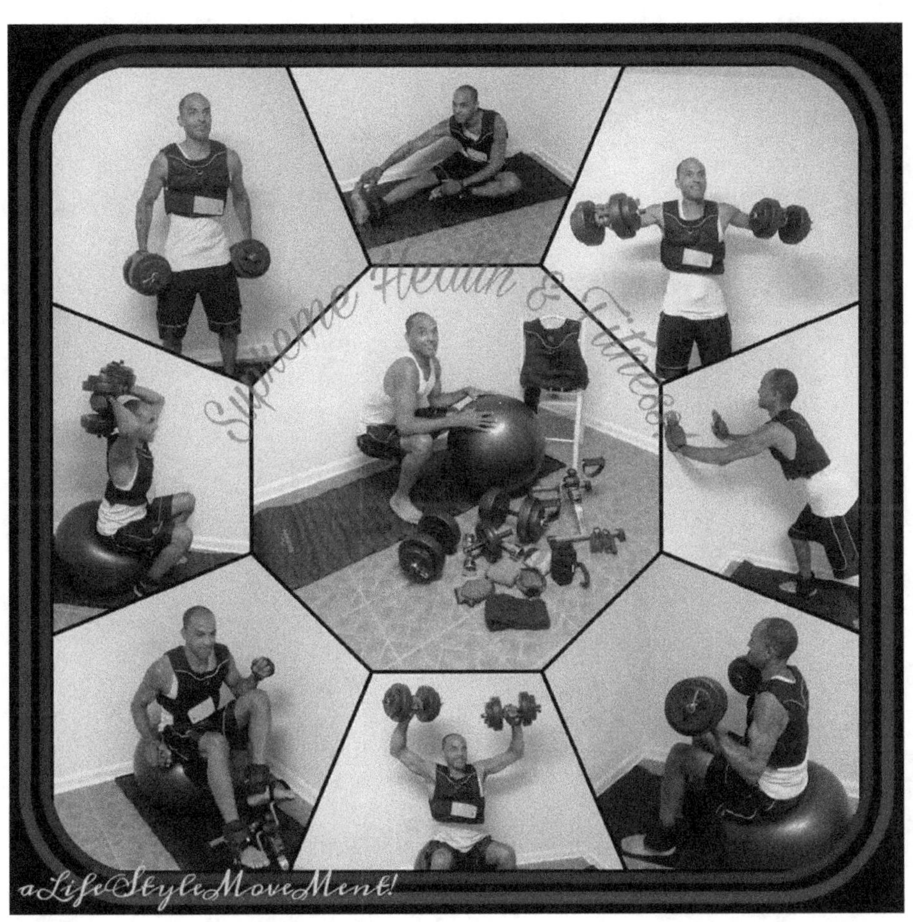
aLifeStyleMoveMent!

Increasing Resistance

=

Increasing Gains

High Resistance Training!

It is very Easy to Increase our Gains At Home … Using the same Activities we just used! From Stretching to Squats – by adding a Weight Vest, Ankle and Wrist Weights and Hand Weights we can Safely Increase Resistance and Successfully Improving Ourselves = Building Your God-Body!

From Head to Feet, we can Increase Our Power, Energy, Health and Wellness!!!!

ALL IN THE COMFORT OF YOUR OWN HOME!!!!

*High Resistance Supreme Stretching!

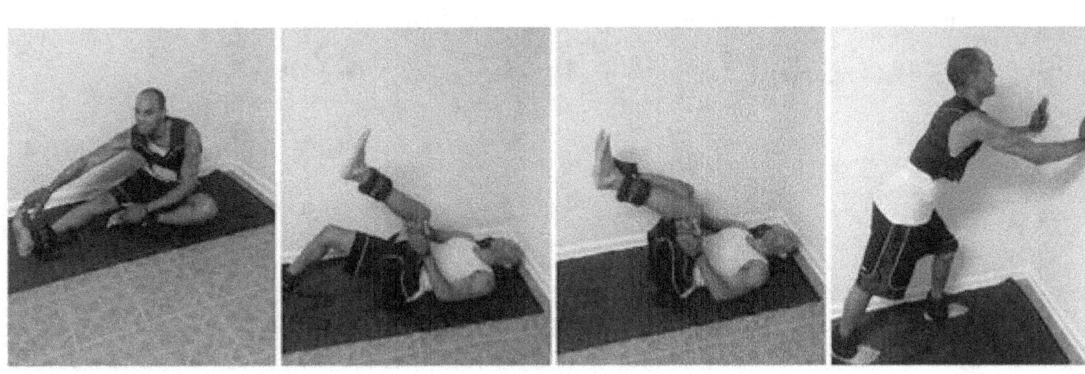

*****

*High Resistance Supreme Aerobics!

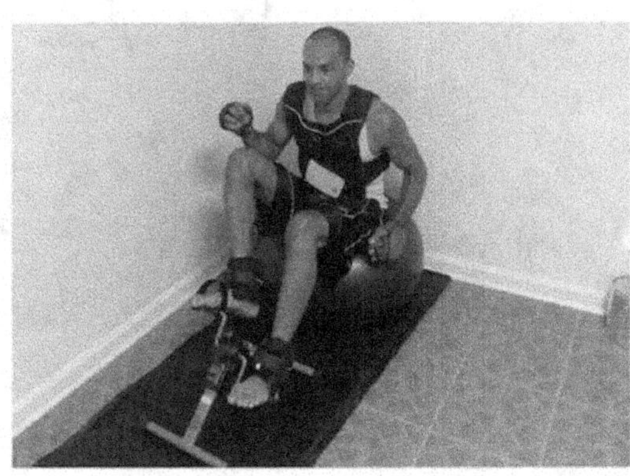
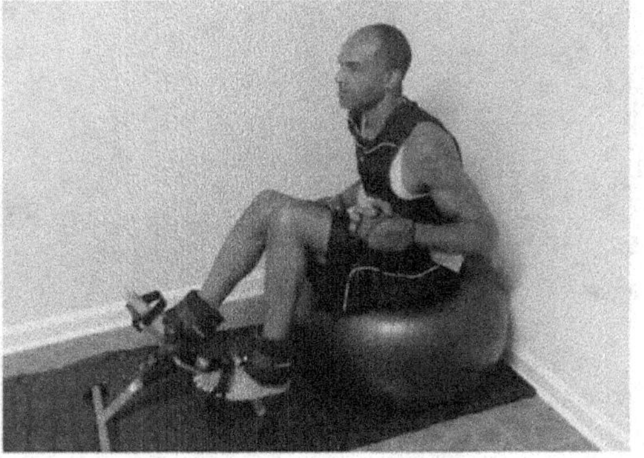

*High Resistance Supreme Pull-Ups!

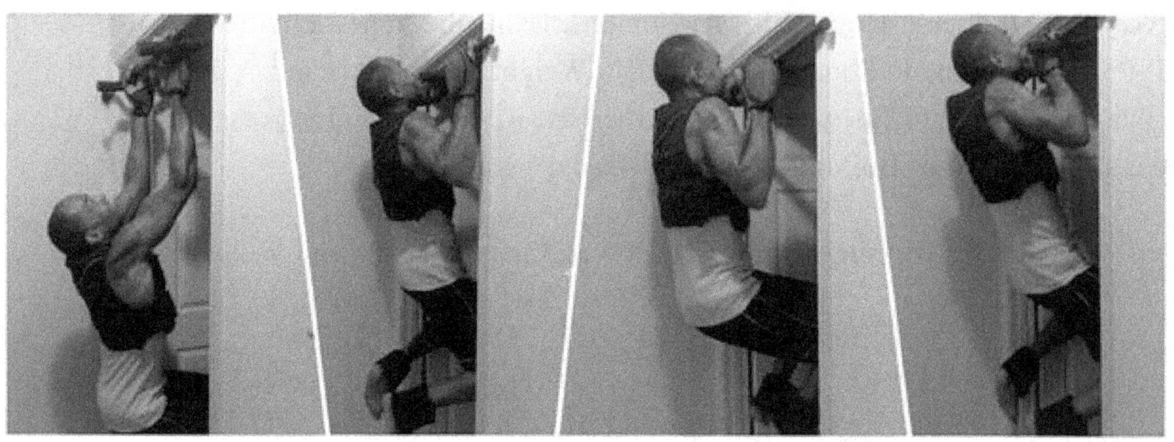

*Each of the 4 Supreme Pull-Ups Grips are displayed: 1. Supreme Under-Hand Grip; 2. Supreme Over-Hand Wide Grip; 3. Supreme Hammer Grip; 4. Supreme Over-Hand Close Grip.

*****

*High Resistance Supreme Bicep Curls

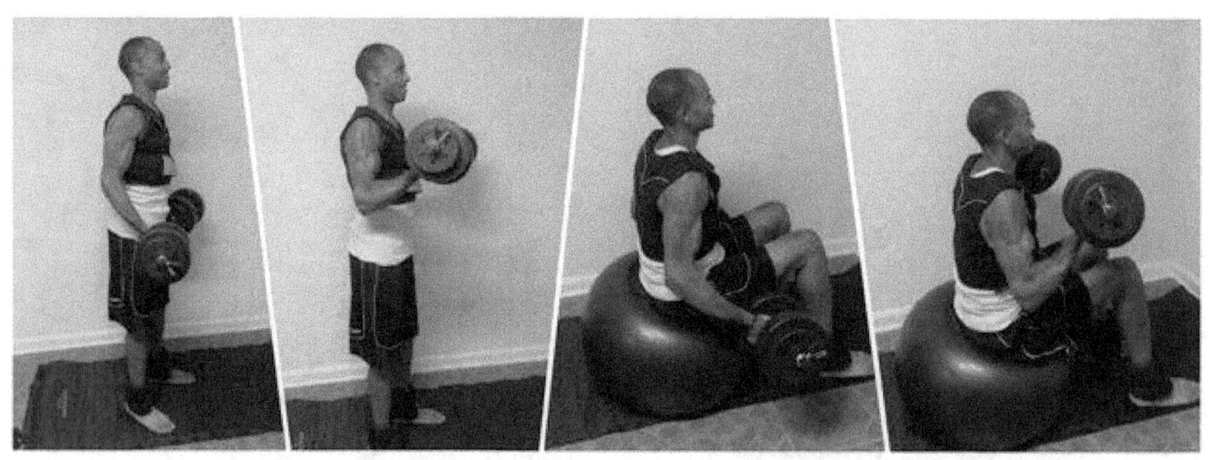

*****

*High Resistance Supreme Shoulder Press

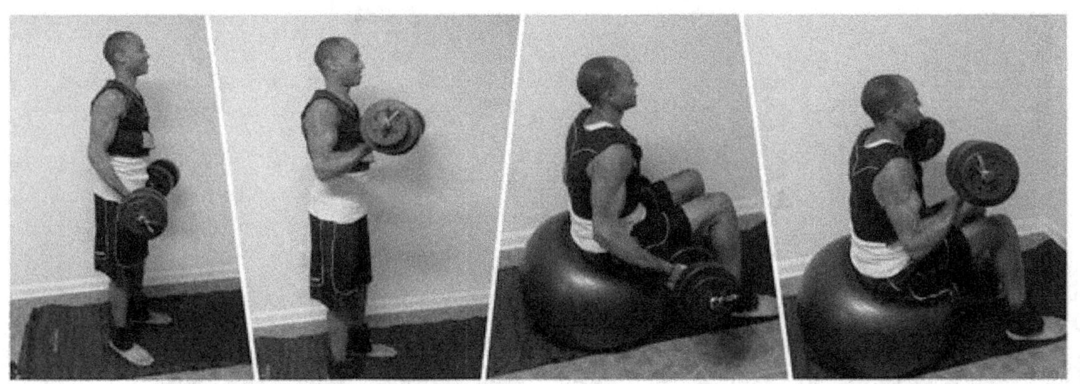

*****

*High Resistance Supreme Shoulder Curls!

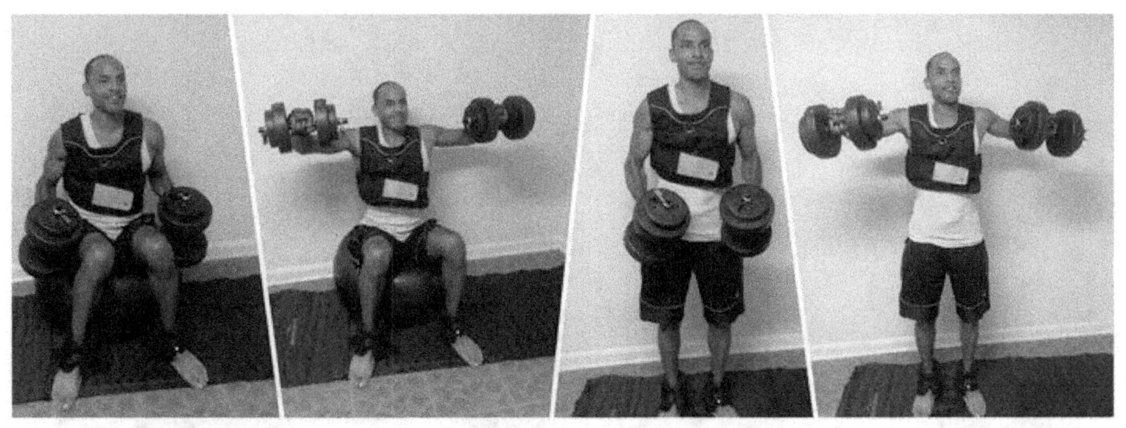

*****

*High Resistance Supreme Back Arms Curl

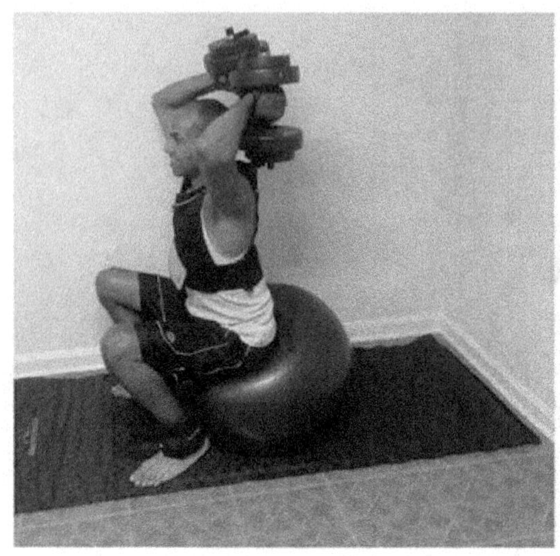 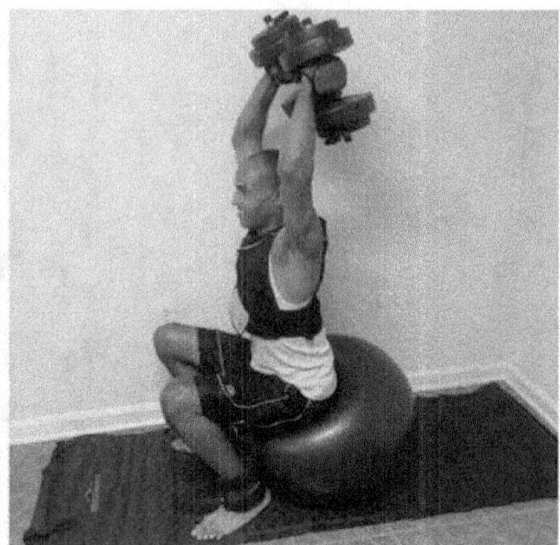

*****

*High Resistance Supreme Squats and Lunges!

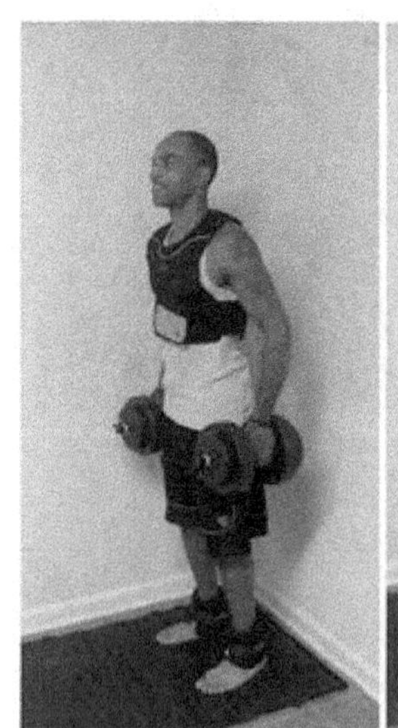 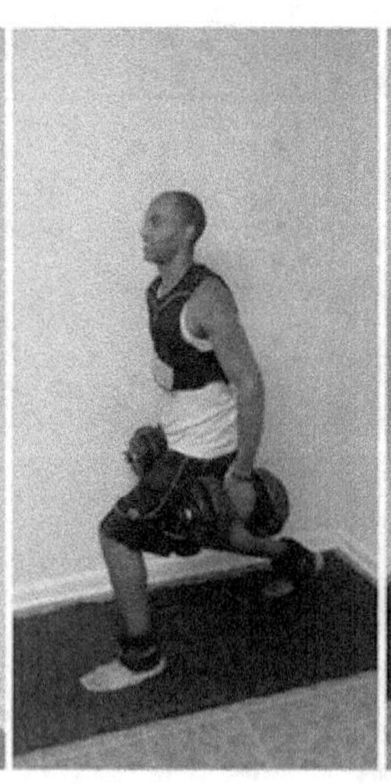 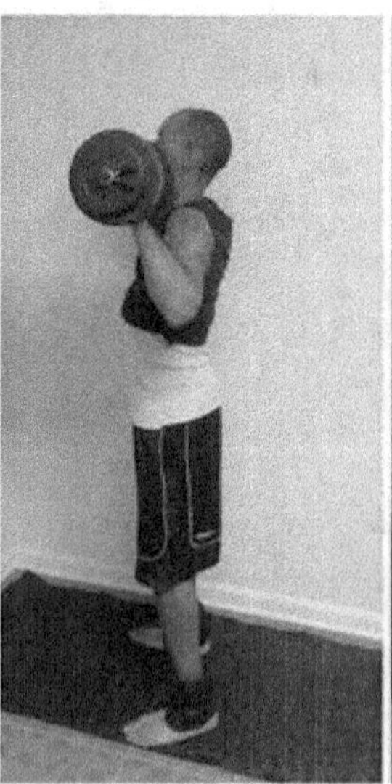 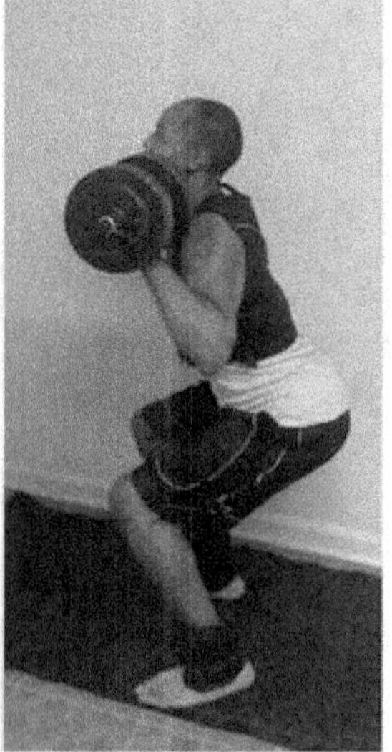

*****

*High Resistance Supreme Step-Ups!

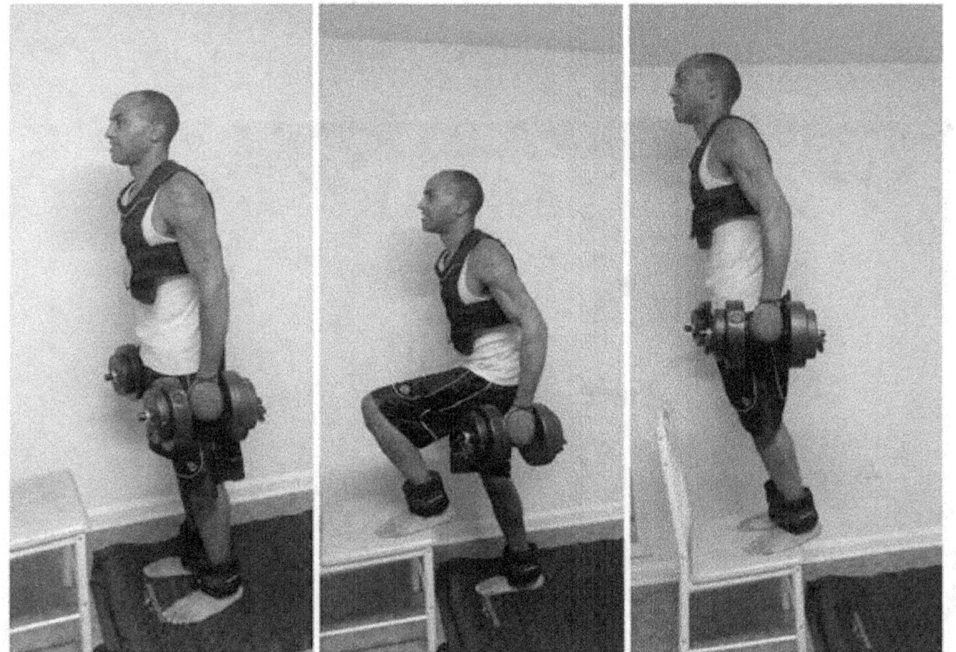

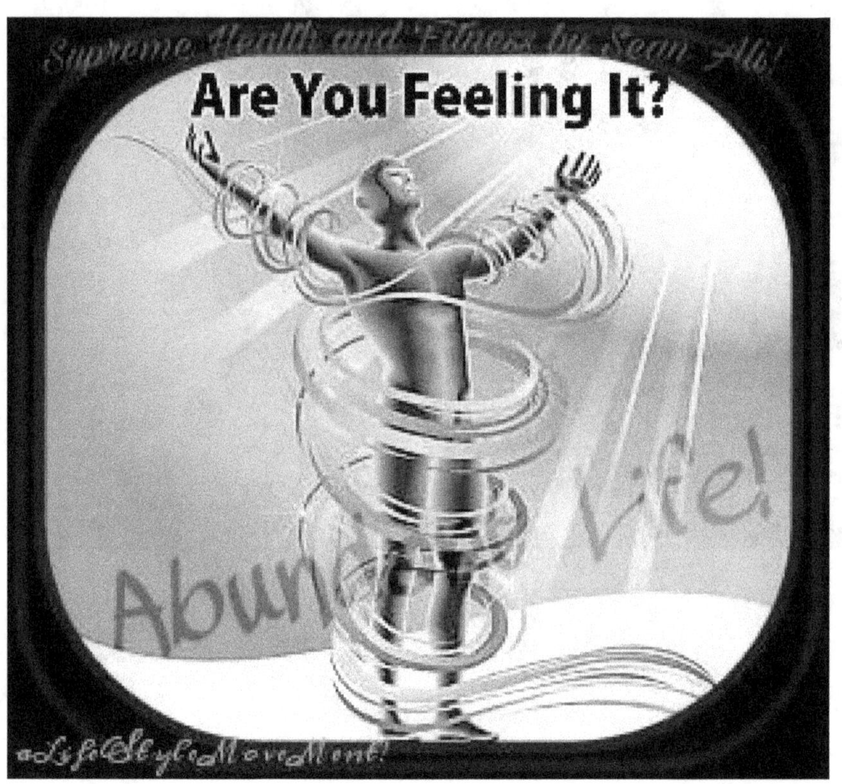
Supreme Health and Fitness by Sean Ali!
Are You Feeling It?
Abundant Life!
aLifeStyleMoveMent!

Conclusion ..... Making Informed Decisions

*****

You are the Direct Express Image & Likeness of The CREATOR!!!!!

Our Bodies ARE Temples of The Most High!!!

We have been Created to LIVE FOREVER!!!

From our Immune System to our Respiratory System, we have an Automatic System that works around the clock to keep us Healthy, Youthful and Alive - Homeostasis! The ONLY reason we fail to Be Healthy, Keep our Youth and Stay Alive is our mis-use and mis-understanding of this Awesome Vehicle we call the Human Body!

At the Root of a Healthy Cardio, Respiratory and Immune System is EXERCISE or Physical Activities!

The Solution to the Fountain Of YOUTH is intricately related to EXERCISE or Physical Activities!

The Foundation for Creating the God-Body to Successfully carry You into the Enjoyment of Abundant LIFE is established through EXERCISE or Physical Activities!

Exercise is like Charging up a Battery that is low on Energy. Exercise Improves the Electrical Current of our Pace-Maker in our Hearts – Improvement in Blood Pressure and Flow. We NEED our Hearts to continuously Beat in order to maintain Life! Exercise is the Best Medicine for our Hearts!

A physically active life begins in childhood, but if you have been unfortunate to not have been as Active as you could have as a child....NO WORRIES...... Even if you did not start early, you can start late. Light to moderate exercise will improve your health at any age - for example, like mall-walking, dancing, t'ai chi, or fitness classes designed for older people.

IT'S NEVER TOO LATE!!!!

AND IT'S VERY EASY!!!!

PLEASE, Continue to exercise as you are Right Now as well as you continue to age. You'll have a healthier heart and fitter body. Exercise can reduce blood pressure, make your joints more flexible, and increase muscular strength and **endurance**. Not only your body benefits: You will improve your mood and your cognitive functions as well.

Keeping your balance as you age is a major issue. Falls that a young person bounces back from can incapacitate or be fatal for older people. Falls in old age are usually the result of poor balance, and keeping fit improves balance.

It may take a bit more initiative, especially if your job is desk-bound, but you will be healthier if you create a personal program of physical activity and exercise after college.

Choose activities you like; you are more likely to stick with them throughout your life.

There are some simple ways to make a difference in your daily physical activity:

- Walk to work, at least part of the way.

- Use the stairs, not the elevator.

- Walk during lunchtime.

- Ride a bicycle.

To be more serious about it, you can exercise at home, join a fitness club, or use the exercise facilities in your office building.

If you like to exercise at home, you can buy barbells and hand weights for resistance training, and for aerobic exercise, use a rowing machine, stationary bike, treadmill, stair climber, or cross-country ski machine. A great way to decide whether these are the best pieces of equipment to purchase for home use is to try them out at a fitness club before buying them.

If you like the social aspects of belonging to a fitness club or find it more motivating, by all means join one, but look before you leap.

Steps in Decision Making

After reading this book you should realize that many decisions are necessary for beginning and maintaining a healthy lifestyle. To make good decisions, you can use the following procedures. These procedures apply to any of life's decisions, not merely those dealing with a healthy lifestyle (**Lab 11-1 and 11-2**):

1.   **Identify and clarify the problem.** You must recognize that a problem exists. Some may simply be annoyances, while others are big issues.

2.   **Gather information.** Learn more about the problem situation. Look for possible causes and solutions.

3.   **Evaluate the evidence.** How accurate is the information? Is it fact or opinion?

4.   **Consider alternatives and implications.** Draw conclusions, then weigh the advantages and disadvantages of each alternative.

5.   **Choose and implement the best alternative.**

Exercise Myths or Misconceptions

Misconceptions exist about what is exercise fact and what is exercise fiction. Here are some common exercise-related fallacies:

■   Passive muscle stimulators expend energy from the electrical outlet in the wall, not from your cells. The energy expended to bring about fat loss must be from within your body.

■   Taking a pill to bring about instant changes in fitness is an illusion. Fitness takes time and effort. The body systems (muscular, cardiovascular, and skeletal) become stronger in response to regular physical activity.

■   **Cellulite** is not something a health gadget or cream can eliminate. Rapid gain or loss of body fat causes the dimpled look associated with the term *cellulite*.

Cellulite: Adipose tissue surrounded by stretched connective tissue.

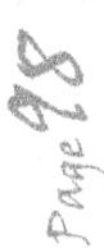

■   Shake, rattle, or roll your fat—it won't disappear. The *only* way to reduce body fat is to use more energy than you consume in calories.

■   Wearing rubberized suits, extra layers of clothing, or working out in a hot environment loses water, not fat. It takes a great deal of heat to melt fat. Such heat would melt the rest of you as well.

■   If spot reduction worked, everyone who chewed gum or talked a lot would have a narrow face.

■   Exercise does not turn fat cells into muscle cells, nor does inactivity turn muscle cells into fat. They are different types of cells. Eat too much and be inactive, and you will enlarge (**hypertrophy**) the fat cells in your body and shrink (**atrophy**) the muscle cells. Eat right and exercise to do the reverse.

■   Rubbing lotions on the skin to lose fat, firm up muscles, or remove lactic acid does not work. Resistance training firms up muscles.

■   Eating extra protein to build stronger muscles doesn't work. Eat more protein than your body uses and the extra will be stored by your body as fat. Increased muscle size comes through resistance training.

■   Losing inches is not necessarily loss of fat. It can also be loss of water or lean muscle tissue.

■   Exercise is only tiring momentarily. It then makes you feel more energetic as you become more fit.

■   In women, resistance training mainly increases muscle strength, not size.

■   Drinking liquids during exercise does not cause **cramping**. Room temperature water (we are 75% Water … NOT soda, juice or any other liquid) should be consumed before, during, and after exercising to replace lost fluids.

Hypertrophy: Enlargement of fat or muscle.

Atrophy: Shrinkage of fat or muscle.

Cramping: Muscular tightness and abdominal or limb pain from dehydration and high body temperature.

Identifying Fitness Misinformation and Quackery

Some advertisers claim—without evidence—that their fitness products offer a quick, easy way to shape up, keep fit, and lose weight. There is no such thing as a no-work, no-sweat way to a healthy, fit body. To get the benefit, you have to do the work.

Watch for these and other warning signs:

- If the claim sounds too good to be true, it probably is.

- If a product really worked, you would see it in headlines, not just in ads.

- The ads claim the product treats a wide range of ailments.

- The information given is unclear, vague, and highly emotional.

- Changes are promised to be quick, dramatic, or miraculous.

- Results are promised to be easy, effortless, guaranteed, or permanent.

- The ads claim relief from conditions for which there are few treatments and no cures.

- The promoter blames problems on a build up of toxins in the body.

- Ads declare the medical community to be against the discovery.

- The ads rely on a guru, testimonials, case histories, and before-and-after photos.

- Products are sold door-to-door, in fliers, through pop-up ads, or by mail order and television advertisements.

- The promoter uses high-pressure sales tactics, one-time-only deals, recruitment for a pyramid sales organization, or demands for large advance payments or long-term contracts.

The next time you watch a TV commercial or see a flyer for a quick weight-loss program, take a moment to consider it. What is being said to you? Who is saying it? In today's day and age we find that to be healthy consumers we need to be educated consumers. The next time you see one of these ads, take a minute to answer the following questions:

■   What claim is being made on behalf of this product?

■   Who is making this claim? Is it an outside source or the company that makes the product?

■   Is everything a testimony about how miraculous the product is?

■   Does the ad list any studies that have been done to demonstrate the product's effectiveness?

■   If yes, is this a credible source?

■   Does it seem like a miracle cure or solution?

■   How does it make you feel that ineffective or dangerous products may be marketed without any sound research?

You can find information on just about everything on the Internet. Of course, not all Internet sites are created equal. Some present research and information, some are trying to sell a product, and some are flat-out misinformation. Here are some suggestions on how to decide whether the information you find is quality and reputable:

1.   **Check for the creator of the site.** It is important to be able to identify whom the authors or creators of the site are. The author should include his or her credentials to demonstrate his or her training and expertise in the subject matter. If this information is missing, be cautious.

2.   **Check the URL.** Website addresses that end with .edu are material from an educational or research institution. Those ending in .gov are government sources. Those ending with .com or .biz are commercial sites generally intended to sell a product. Because the content of websites is not monitored for accuracy, you may be reading inaccurate, biased, misleading, partial, or false information. This is much more likely to occur on commercial sites than on any other type of website. In addition, if the URL includes a personal name, the site may simply be an individual creating a forum for his or her personal opinion.

3.   **Check for advertising.** Websites often accept advertising to help pay the cost of maintaining the site. If the products being advertised are the same as or related to the nature of the information you seek, be cautious. You'd hate to rely on information that has been biased so as not to offend or upset an advertiser. When that happens, you can be certain the information you are viewing is misleading.

4.   **Look for accuracy.** Be on the lookout for sites that integrate personal opinions, testimonials, or leading statements about the material you are searching for. Do not assume the first site you visit has accurate information. Gather information from several sites on the same topic and look for common themes. Sites that go into greater depth with their information (as opposed to stating one "fact" and then presenting opinion afterward) are more likely to be accurate. Always back up data from Internet sources with other forms of information to make your data gathering more comprehensive and, in turn, more accurate.

5.   **Look for timeliness.** Websites should always contain "updated on" dates to indicate when the information was created. If these dates are missing, you should find additional sources to support the materials' timeliness. Some websites are created but then never updated, and there is no systematic removal of old sites from the Internet.

In addition, many sites contain links to other websites or other information. If many of the links are no longer available or contain outdated material, exercise caution regarding what you find. Make certain you find supporting materials from other sources.

Selecting a Fitness Professional Who Is Right for You

•	Is the fitness professional's workspace convenient to your workplace or home, or is training available in your home?

•	Are new clients provided with a pre-exercise screening for health risk factors, and is a fitness program designed specifically for their needs?

•	Does the fitness professional offer the expertise, programs, and services you need to achieve your fitness goals?

References

American College of Sports Medicine (ACSM). *ACSM's Guidelines for Exercise Testing and Prescription*. Philadelphia: Lippincott Williams & Wilkins, 2006.

American College of Sports Medicine (ACSM). ACSM position stand: The recommended quantity and quality of exercise for developing and maintaining cardiorespiratory, muscular fitness and flexibility in healthy adults. *Medicine and Science in Sports and Exercise* 1998; 30:975–991.

ACSM. Quantity and Quality of Exercise for Developing and Maintaining Cardiorespitory, Musculoskeletal, and Neuromotor Fitness in Apparently Healthy Adults: Guidance for Prescribing Exercise. *Medicine and Science in Sports and Exercise*. DOI: 10.1249/MSS.0b0138213fefb

American Heart Association. Cholesterol. http://www.heart.org/HEARTORG/Conditions/Cholesterol/Cholesterol_UCM_001089_SubHomePage.jsp. Accessed September 25, 2011.

American Heart Association. Diabetes mellitus. http://www.heart.org/HEARTORG/Conditions/Diabetes/Diabetes_UCM_001091_SubHomePage.jsp. Accessed September 25, 2011.

- Resting heart rate. 2004c. http://www.heart.org/HEARTORG/ [June 14, 2004].

- Target heart rate. 2004d. http://www.heart.org/HEARTORG/ [June 14, 2004].

American Heart Association (AHA). A statement on exercise: Benefits and recommendations for physical activity programs for all Americans. *Circulation* 1995; 91:580.

Blair S. N. and Jackson A. S. Physical fitness and activity as separate heart disease risk factors: A meta-analysis. *Medicine and Science in Sports and Exercise* 2001; 33:762–764.

Borg G. A. Psychophysical basis of perceived exertion. *Medicine and Science in Sports and Exercise* 1982; 14:377.

Carroll J. F. and Kyser C. K. Exercise training in obesity lowers blood pressure independent of weight change. *Medicine and Science in Sports and Exercise* 2002; 34:596–601.

Cooper K. H. *The Aerobics Program for Well-Being*. Toronto: Bantam Books, 1982.

Erikssen G. Physical fitness and changes in mortality: The survival of the fittest. *Sports Medicine* 2001; 31:571–576.

Fletcher G., et al. American Heart Association: Statement on exercise. *Circulation* 1992; 86:726.

Garber C. E., Blissmer B., Deschenes M. R., Franklin B. A., Lamonte M. J., Lee I-M., Nieman D. C., and Swain D. P. Quantity and Quality of Exercise for Developing and Maintaining Cardiorespiratory, Musculoskeletal, and Neuromotor Fitness in Apparently Healthy Adults: Guidance for Prescribing Exercise. *Medicine in Science and Sports and Exercise* 2011; 43(7): 1334–1359,

Myers J., Prakash M., Froelicher V., Do D., Partington S., and Atwood J. E. Exercise capacity and mortality among men referred for exercise testing. *New England Journal of Medicine* 2002; 346:793–801.

Haskell W. L., Lee I. M., Pate R. R., Powell K. E., Blair S. N., Franklin B. A., Macera C. A., Heath G. W., Thompson P. D., and Bauman A. American College of Sports Medicine, American Heart Association. Physical activity and public health: Updated recommendation for adults from the American College of Sports Medicine and the American Heart Association. *Circulation* 2007; 116(9):1081–1093. http://circ.ahajournals.org/content/116/9/1081.full.pdf

Public Health Service. *Surgeon General's Report on Physical Activity and Health*. Washington, DC: U.S. Government Printing Office, 1996.

UC Davis Health System. The well-connected report: Exercise. March 2000. http://www.ucdmc.ucdavis.edu/healthconsumers/health/wellconnected/exercise29.html [June 14, 2004].

U.S. DHHS. *2008 Physical Activity Guidelines for Americans*. www.health.gov/paguidelines.

————. Prescription of resistance training for health and disease. *Medicine and Science in Sports and Exercise* 1999; 31:38–45.

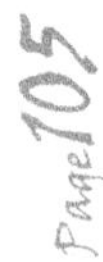

American College of Sports Medicine (ACSM). The recommended quantity and quality of exercise for developing and maintaining cardiorespiratory and muscular fitness and flexibility in healthy adults. *Medicine and Science in Sports and Exercise* 1998; 30:975–991.

American College of Sports Medicine. Quantity and Quality of Exercise for Developing and Maintaining Cardiorespiratory, Musculoskeletal, and Neuromotor Fitness in Apparently Healthy Adults: Guidance for Prescribing Exercise. *Medicine and Science in Sports and Exercise.* DOI: 10.1249/MSS.0b0138213fefb

Braill P. A., et al. Muscular strength and physical function. *Medicine and Science in Sports and Exercise* 2000; 32:412–416.

Ebben W. P. and Jensen R. L. Strength training for women. *Physician and Sports Medicine* 1998; 26:86.

Feigenbaum M. S. and Pollock M. L. Strength training: Rationale for current guidelines for adult fitness programs. *Physician and Sports Medicine* 1997; 25:44.

Garber, C. E., et al. Quantity and quality of exercise for developing and maintaining cardiorespiratory, musculoskeletal, and neuromotor fitness in apparently healthy adults: Guidance for prescribing exercise. *Medicine in Science and Sports and Exercise* 2011; 43(7):1334–1359.

National Safety Council. *Inquiry Facts.* Itasca, IL: National Safety Council, 2007.

Stamford B. Weight training basics. Part 1: Choosing the best options. *Physician and Sports Medicine* 1998; 26:115–116.

Sean Ali

Understanding Carbohydrates: LIFE Energy, Fiber, Sugar and Starch! (Science Of LIFE Series)

ISBN-13: 978-1520559988, **ISBN-10:** 1520559984

#1 New Release in Fiber

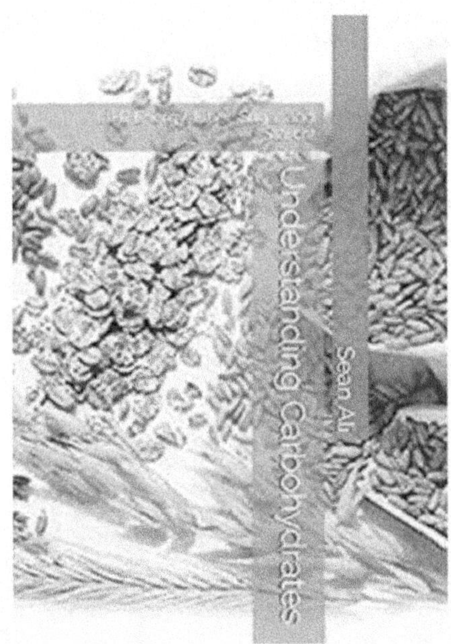

Project Summary
OxyGen!: The Breath Of LIFE In Atomic Form!
Authored by Sean Ali, Authored by Kareem Tyree, Authored by Gabriella Monique, Authored by Khlail Malik

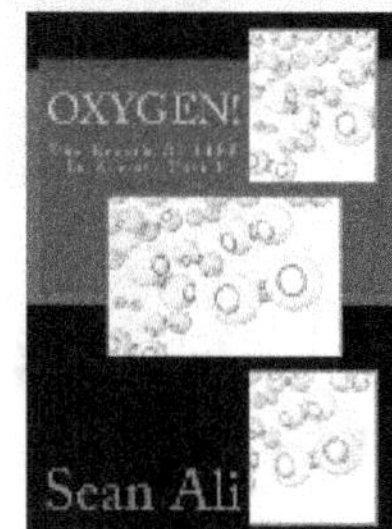

List Price: **$35.00**

7" x 10" (17.78 x 25.4 cm)
Full Color on White paper
182 pages

ISBN-13: **978-1548589561** (CreateSpace-Assigned)
ISBN-10: **154858956X**
BISAC: Medical / Healing

Peace and Blessings of Health!

*Do YOU have health issues that YOU want to over-come?

*Do YOU want to Improve the Quality of YOUR Life?

*Do YOU want to achieve ABUNDANT LIFE?

*** THEN THIS BOOK IS FOR YOU!! ***

Oxygen IS the Breath Of LIFE in Atomic form!

This short work is a composition of Scientific, Medical and Spiritually based research , compiled into a comprehensive, easily read and understood format, designed to Help the reader achieve and maintain their own Supreme Health and Fitness!

We have 3 major functions - Eating, Drinking and Breathing, that must be performed in order for us to be considered Alive......... Of these 3 functions, Breathing is the least explored, taught or performed properly - BUT THE MOST IMPORTANT.

We can go 7-10 days without Food before signs of Nutritional deficiency. We can go 3-7 days without Water before we present symptoms........ But, 1 Minute of Oxygen deprivation/deficiency causes Cellular Damage!

Our Cells need 2 elements for Growth and Reproduction = OXYGEN & GLUCOSE !

Let's explore and discover the Amazing Power of Oxygen and the Natural Abilty to Heal Self!

OXYGEN IS THE BREATH OF LIFE IN ATOMIC FORM !

OPEN THIS BOOK - and take the steps to Successfully Build Your own Supreme Health & Fitness!

PEACE!

CreateSpace eStore: https://www.createspace.com/7316042

Project Summary
LIFE Energy!: *The Sun, Gluceose & WHY Humans Are Herbivores!
Authored by Sean Ali, Authored by Kareem Tyree, Authored by Gabriella Monique, Authored by Khalil Malik

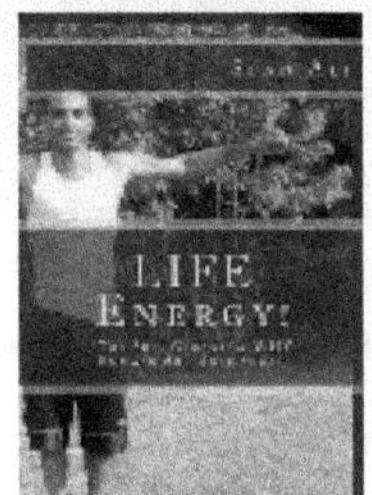

List Price: **$32.00**

7" x 10" (17.78 x 25.4 cm)
Full Color on White paper
166 pages

ISBN-13: 978-1548545017 (CreateSpace-Assigned)
ISBN-10: 1548545015
BISAC: Health & Fitness / Healthy Living

Peace and Blessings of Health!

*Do YOU have a health issue that YOU would like to over-come?
*Do YOU want to Improve the Quality of YOUR Life?
*Do YOU want to experience ABUNDANT LIFE?

*** OPEN THIS BOOK - NOW!!! ***

This small book is written with the purpose of re-examining the role of Nutrition in health care and everyday Life......LIFE IS ENERGY.....Nutrition is a descriptive term to describe how we replenish our Life Energy.
Understanding Nutrition is the equivalent of understanding Energy and Knowledge of Nutrition enables us to make precise Energy adjustments through Nutrients to provide the proper Energy needed for all our body functions/tasks – from achieving Homeostasis, facilitating our Growth, Development and Self- Healing.
We come from the Earth and all our Solutions are manifested from the Earth...... All we have to do is return back to the Earth and extract what we need.
Food is our naturally occurring vehicle, perfectly designed for administering the Life Energy in the form of Nutrition.
Our Food choices and the Energy released from it, presents as either the root cause of our dis-ease or the base for our Solution.
From our Cells to our Immune system, we are Created to Heal and Regenerate Self with the aide of proper Nutrition/Energy.
Our Food is our Medicine ONLY with proper application...... There is no in-between, which means that we are either eating to die – OR – Eating To LIVE !!!!
Energy is the Key to LIFE and we Know that the Sun is the Source of all Energy, so if we focus on how to obtain as much Sun in the form of food as possible = the Key to Nutritional Health and Therapy.
Let us explore and examine Life Energy and how to obtain the best Quality and Value so that we may successfully manifest the Best out of Life and Enjoy a long, active and fruitful Life span!

Achieving and Maintaining Supreme Health and Fitness by increasing the level of Knowledge and Science of Life!

Peace
Sean Ali

CreateSpace eStore: https://www.createspace.com/7310862

Understanding Carb-O-Hydrates!: *Life Energy, Fiber, Glucose & Starch!

Authored by Sean Ali, Authored by Kareem Tyree, Authored by Gabriella Monique, Authored by Khalil Malik

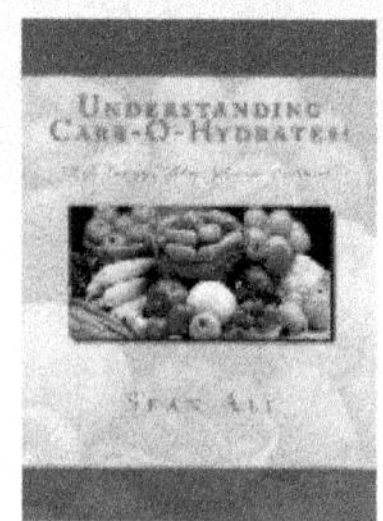

List Price: **$30.00**

7" x 10" (17.78 x 25.4 cm)
Full Color on White paper
158 pages

ISBN-13: **978-1548543143** (CreateSpace-Assigned)
ISBN-10: **1548543144**
BISAC: **Health & Fitness / Healthy Living**

Peace and Blessings of Health!

*Do YOU have health issues that YOU want to over-come?
*Do YOU want to Improve the Quality of YOUR Life?
*Do YOU want to experience ABUNDANT LIFE?

*** THEN THIS BOOK IS FOR YOU!! ***

There is a disproportionate amount of fad diets and food-like TOXIC items that are available and which we are bombarded with that promote a detrimentally 'low' or 'no' Carb meal plan that goes TOTALLY against ALL Nutritional science and evidence of the function of Carbohydrates.

There is little to no serious governmental regulation of these types of claims or food-like items and most are cases of clever advertisement vs actual claims of quality and value.

This small book has been produced to provide understanding of the Nutritional and Life value of Carbohydrates - from a Scientific analogy, while simultaneously shedding light on these false claims and food-like products so that YOU can make the Best Life choices for YOUR successful Growth & Development!

Let us explore and learn about our Primary Energy source and become able to make the best Nutritional choices.

OPEN THIS BOOK - and Begin the steps to Successfully Build and Maintain Your own Supreme Health and Fitness!

Peace !
Sean Ali

CreateSpace eStore: https://www.createspace.com/7310656

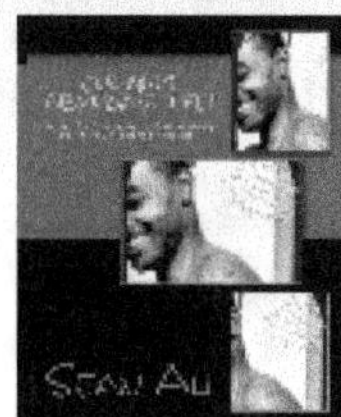

Project Summary

Enjoying Abundant LIFE!: Scientific Concepts to Successfully Build YOUR Supreme Health!
Authored by Sean Ali

List Price: **$35.00**

8" x 10" (20.32 x 25.4 cm)
Full Color on White paper
170 pages

ISBN-13: 978-1546732075 (CreateSpace-Assigned)
ISBN-10: 1546732071
BISAC: Medical / Healing

Peace and Blessings of Health!

*Do YOU have a health issue that YOU would like to over-come?
*Do YOU want to Improve the Quality of YOUR Life?
*Do YOU want to experience ABUNDANT LIFE?

*** OPEN THIS BOOK - NOW!!! ***

This small book is written with the purpose of re-examining the role of Nutrition in health care and everyday Life......LIFE IS
ENERGY.....Nutrition is a descriptive term to describe how we replenish our Life Energy.
Understanding Nutrition is the equivalent of understanding Energy
Knowledge of Nutrition enables us to make precise Energy adjustments through Nutrients to provide the proper Energy
needed for all our body functions/tasks – from achieving Homeostasis, facilitating our Growth, Development and Self-
Healing.
We come from the Earth and all our Solutions are manifested from the Earth...... All we have to do is return back to the
Earth and extract what we need.
Food is our naturally occuring vehicle, perfectly designed for administering the Life Energy in the form of Nutrition.
Our Food choices and the Energy released from it, presents as either the root cause of our dis-ease or the base for our
Solution.
From our Cells to our Immune system, we are Created to Heal and Regenerate Self with the aide of proper
Nutrition/Energy.
Our Food is our Medicine ONLY with proper application...... There is no in-between, which means that we are either eating
to die – OR – Eating To LIVE !!!!
Energy is the Key to LIFE and we Know that the Sun is the Source of all Energy, so if we focus on how to obtain as much
Sun in the form of food as possible = the Key to Nutritional Health and Therapy.
Let us explore and examine Life Energy and how to obtain the best Quality and Value so that we may successfully
manifest the Best out of Life and Enjoy a long, active and fruitful Life-span!

Achieving and Maintaining Supreme Health and Fitness by increasing the level of Knowledge and Science of Life!

Peace
Sean Ali

CreateSpace eStore: https://www.createspace.com/7174743

Project Summary
Understanding Our Human Energy!: Energy Cycle & Transformation to Achieve Abundant LIFE!
Authored by Sean Ali

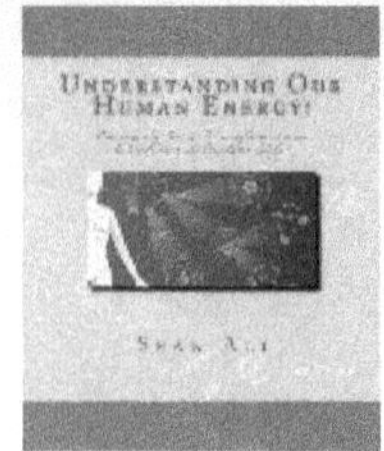

List Price: **$45.00**

8" x 10" (20.32 x 25.4 cm)
Full Color on White paper
224 pages

ISBN-13: 978-1546343462 (CreateSpace-Assigned)
ISBN-10: 1546343466
BISAC: Medical / Alternative Medicine

Peace and Blessings of Life!

•Do YOU Have health ailments/issues that YOU would like to over-come??
•Do YOU want to Improve the Quality of YOUR Life??
•Do YOU want to Experience and Enjoy ABUNDANT LIFE??
** Then this book is for YOU!

This small book is written so that we can explore and gain an Understanding of what our Human Energy System is, with a particular focus on What our Energy is, the Best sources and What to avoid to successfully Grow and LIVE so that we can Enjoy to the fullest, our GOD-Given potential of a Long and Abundant LIFE !!!!!!!!
Understanding our Human Energy is synonymous with Understanding our LIFE...it's what keeps us Alive and the main difference between Us and a body in the grave - Human Energy !!!!
Human Energy is manifested in the form of FOOD....Growing Our Own Food is the ONLY way that ensures we recieve the Highest Quality Life Energy - Straight from the Source!

OPEN THIS BOOK and Begin the neccessary steps to Improve the Quality of YOUR LIFE!

Building and Maintaining Supreme Health & Fitness by increasing the level of Knowledge and Science of Life!

Peace!
Sean Ali, BS Health & Wellness

CreateSpace eStore: https://www.createspace.com/7126564

Project Summary

The Manual Of Healing Herbal Elements!: *Earth-based Solutions for Healing, Health & Life!*
Authored by Sean Ali, Authored by Kareem Tyree, Authored by Gabriella Monique, Authored by Khalil Malik

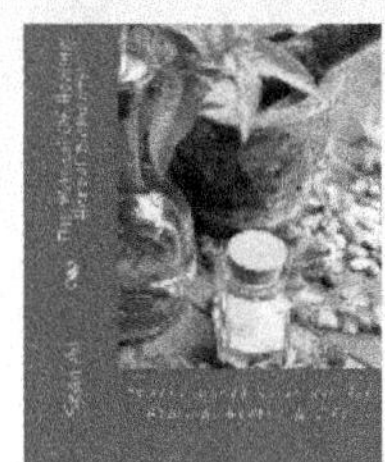

List Price: **$65.00**

8" x 10" (20.32 x 25.4 cm)
Full Color on White paper
336 pages

ISBN-13: **978-1547137985** (CreateSpace-Assigned)
ISBN-10: **1547137983**
BISAC: Medical / Holistic Medicine

Peace and Blessings of Health!
This small work is being presented as a Manual of Healing, Health and Life. A comprehensive and scientific Handbook of Analysis and Research on over 80 Clinically & Commonly accessible Life & Healing Energy Herbal Elements. Each Herbal Element is categorized to include the latest research on the Uses, Actions, Dosages, Client Considerations, Contraindications & Interactions.
As many of Us are witnessing the RISE in Life-threatening dis-eases, especially in childhood Obesity and Diabetes, we are looking for more Natural ways to Heal.
This Manual Of Healing is a Professional Grade handbook to Help YOU choose and use the BEST Naturally occurring Life Elements to Successfully Heal YourSelf!
We come from the Earth and ALL our Solutions come from the Earth!

PEACE!
Sean Ali

CreateSpace eStore: **https://www.createspace.com/7225520**

Understanding & Creating Herbal Healing!: Teas, Decoctions & Tinctures!
Authored by Sean Ali, Authored by Khalil Malik, Authored by Kareem Tyree, Authored by Gabriella Monique

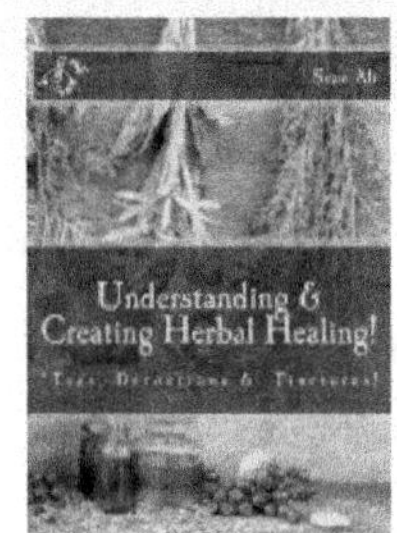

List Price: **$22.00**

7" x 10" (17.78 x 25.4 cm)
Full Color on White paper
108 pages

ISBN-13: 978-1548105457 (CreateSpace-Assigned)
ISBN-10: 1548105457
BISAC: Medical / Healing

Peace and Blessings of Health!

This small work represents Volume 2 of my Science Of Healing Series and is being presented as a Handbook of Healing through the vehicles of Teas, Decoctions and Tinctures.

This is a comprehensive and scientific Handbook of Analysis and Research on over 30 Clinically used & easily accessible Life & Healing Energy Herbal Elements.

This Handbook Of Healing is Professional Grade and designed specifically to Help YOU choose and use the BEST Naturally occurring Life Elements to Successfully Heal YourSelf!
We come from the Earth and ALL our Solutions come from the Earth!

PEACE!
Sean Ali

CreateSpace eStore: https://www.createspace.com/7257513

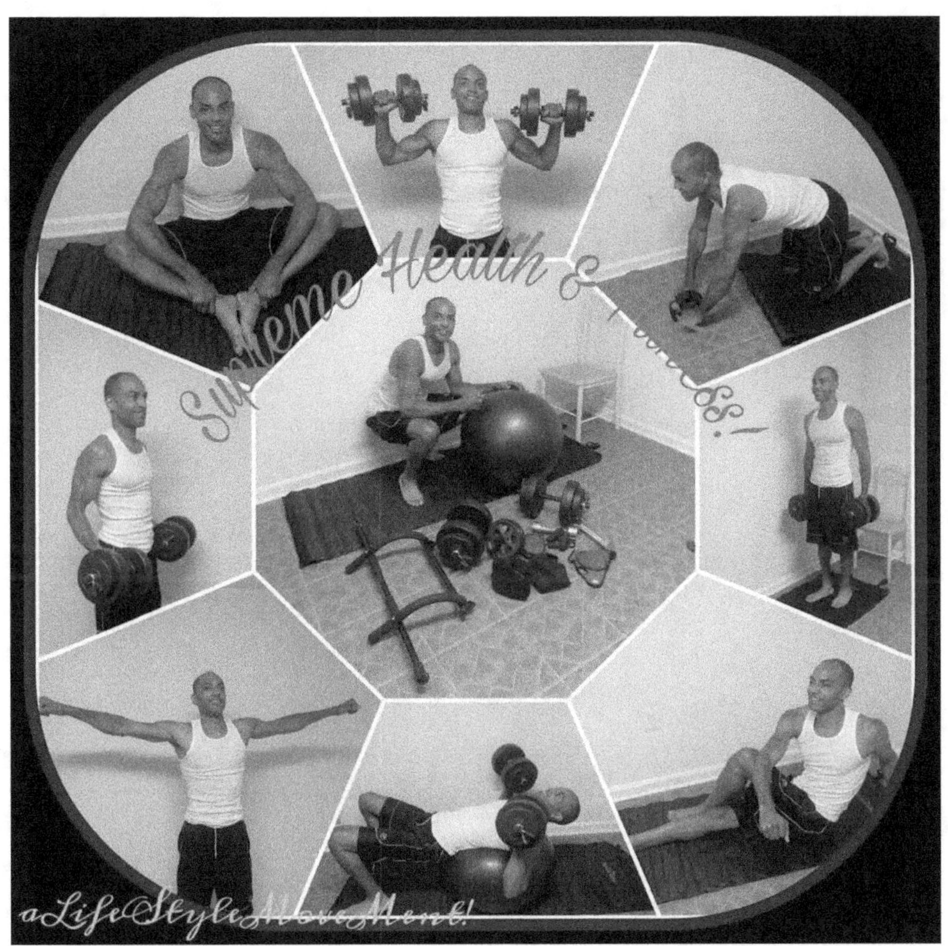
Supreme Health & Fitness!
aLifeStyleMoveMent!

Supreme Health & Fitness by Sean Ali!

Achieving and Maintaining Supreme Health by increasing the level of Knowledge and Science of LIFE!

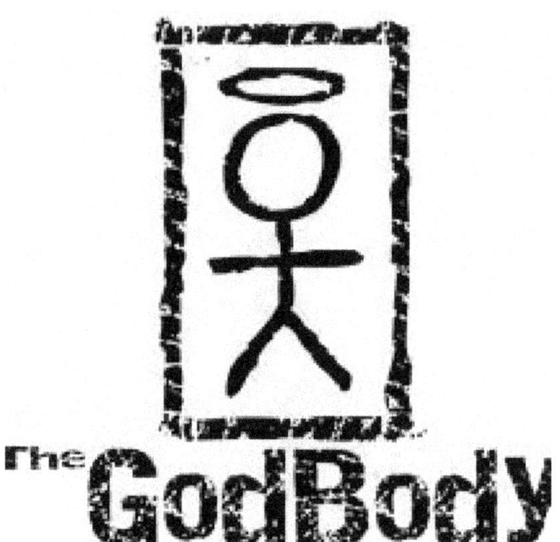

The GodBody

Handbook To Supreme Health & Fitness! ... At-Home Guide to Successfully Build Your God-Body!